this coloring book belongs to:

THIS COLORING BOOK BELONGS TO:

____

50 QUOTES WITH GEOMETRIC BACKGROUND FOR COLORING, ENJOY!!

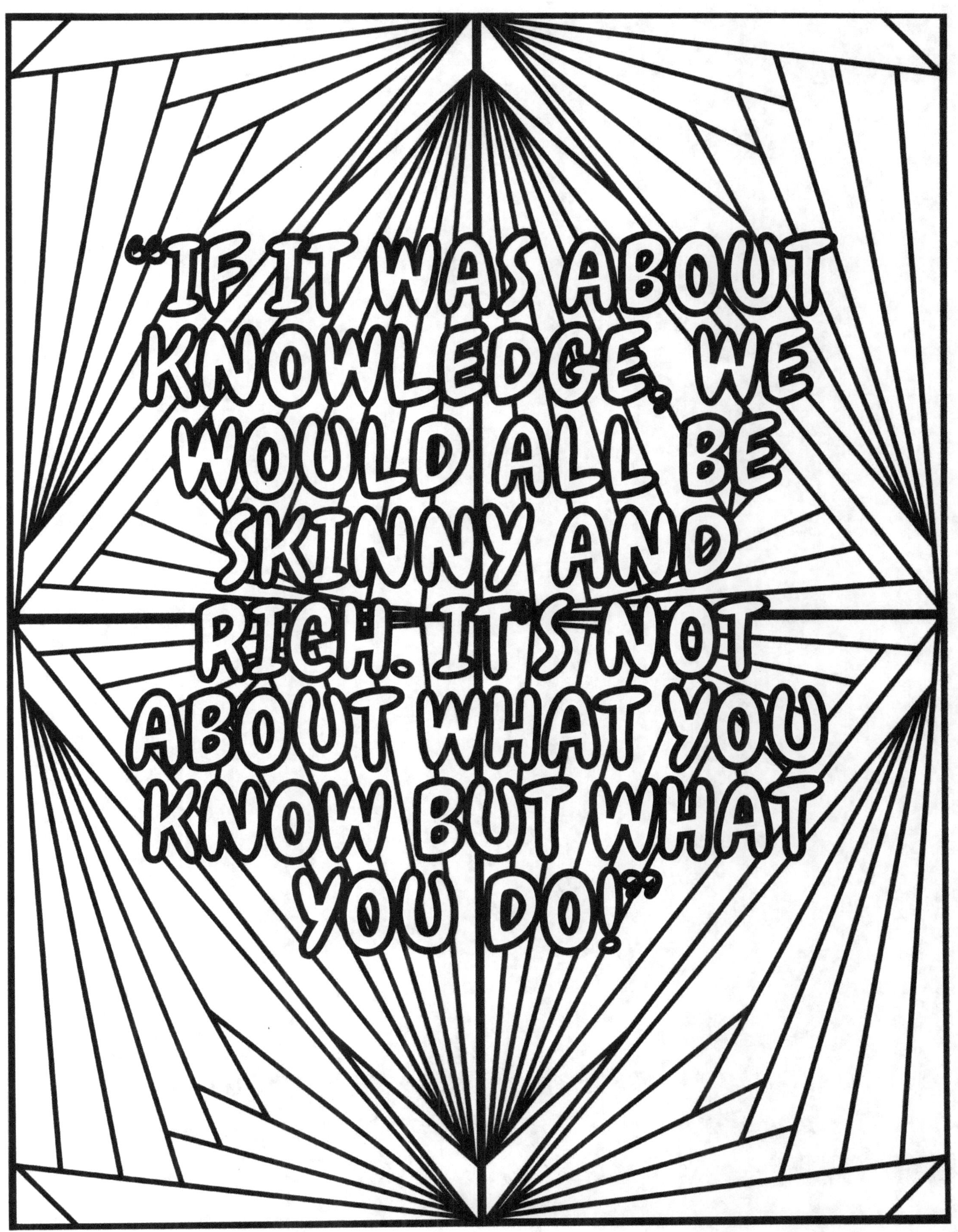

"IF IT WAS ABOUT KNOWLEDGE, WE WOULD ALL BE SKINNY AND RICH. IT'S NOT ABOUT WHAT YOU KNOW BUT WHAT YOU DO!"

"If it was about knowledge, we would all be skinny and rich. It's not about what you know but what you do!"

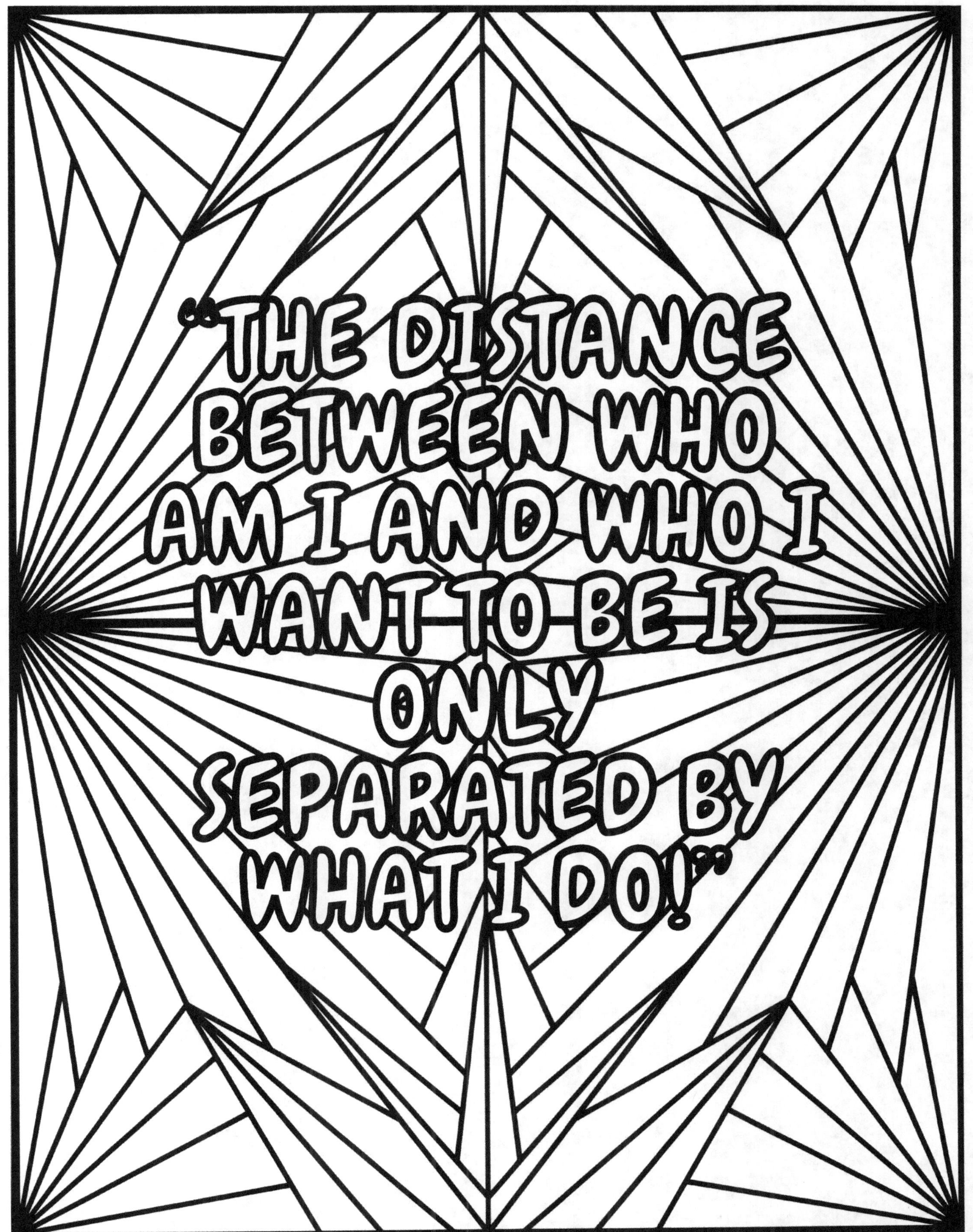

"THE DISTANCE BETWEEN WHO AM I AND WHO I WANT TO BE IS ONLY SEPARATED BY WHAT I DO!"

"The distance between who am I and who I want
to be is only separated by what I do!"

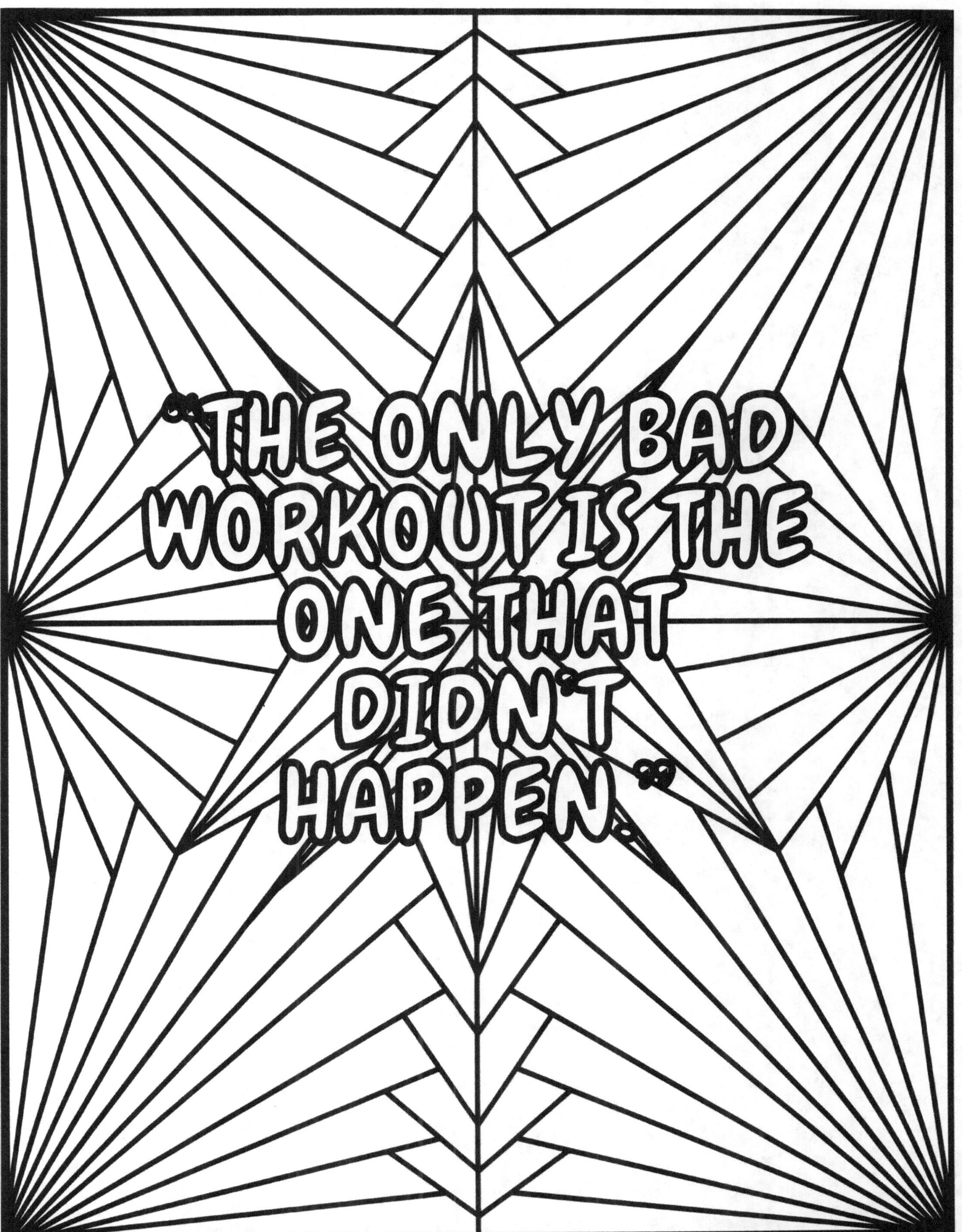
"THE ONLY BAD WORKOUT IS THE ONE THAT DIDN'T HAPPEN."

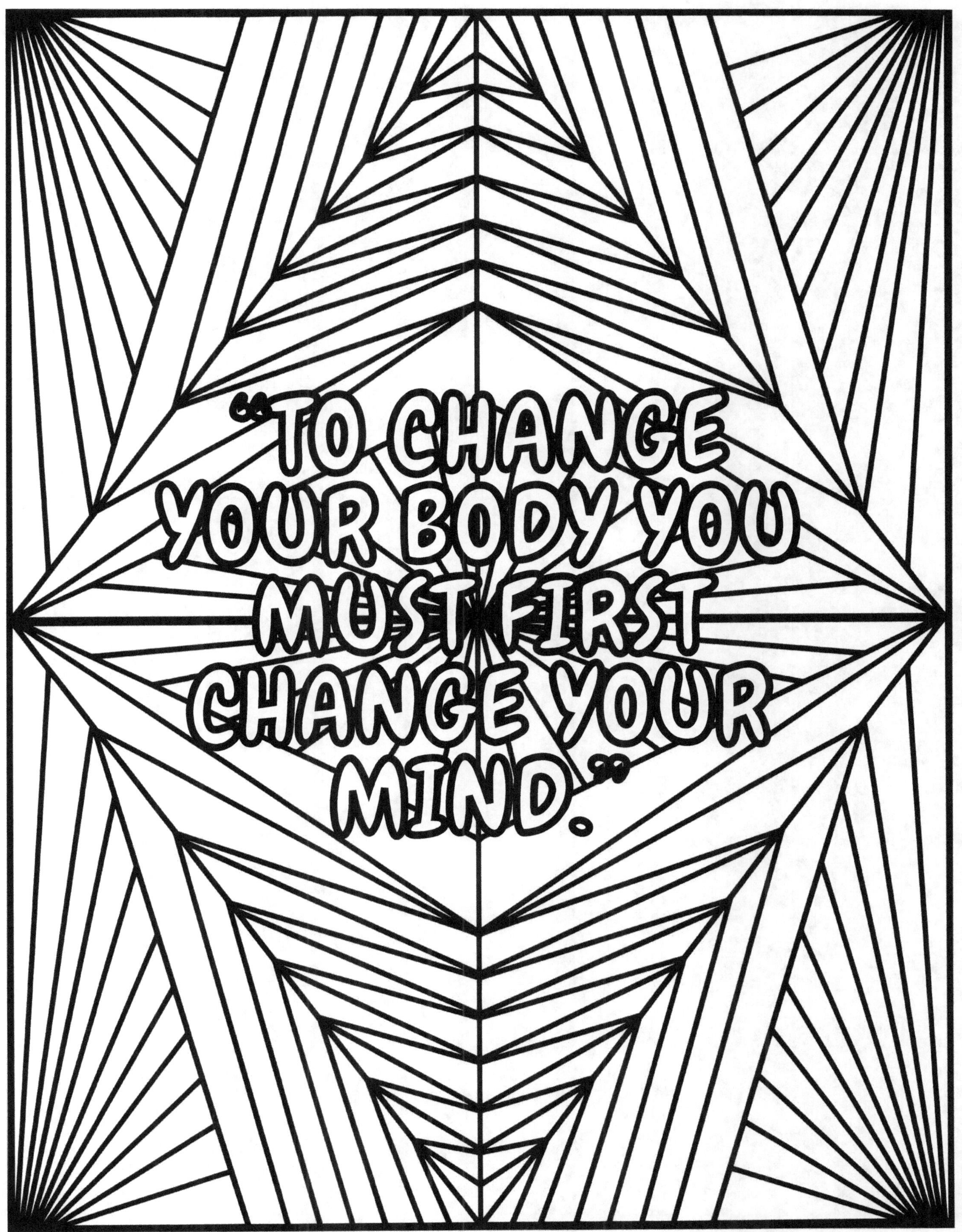

"TO CHANGE YOUR BODY YOU MUST FIRST CHANGE YOUR MIND."

"To change your body you must first
change your mind."

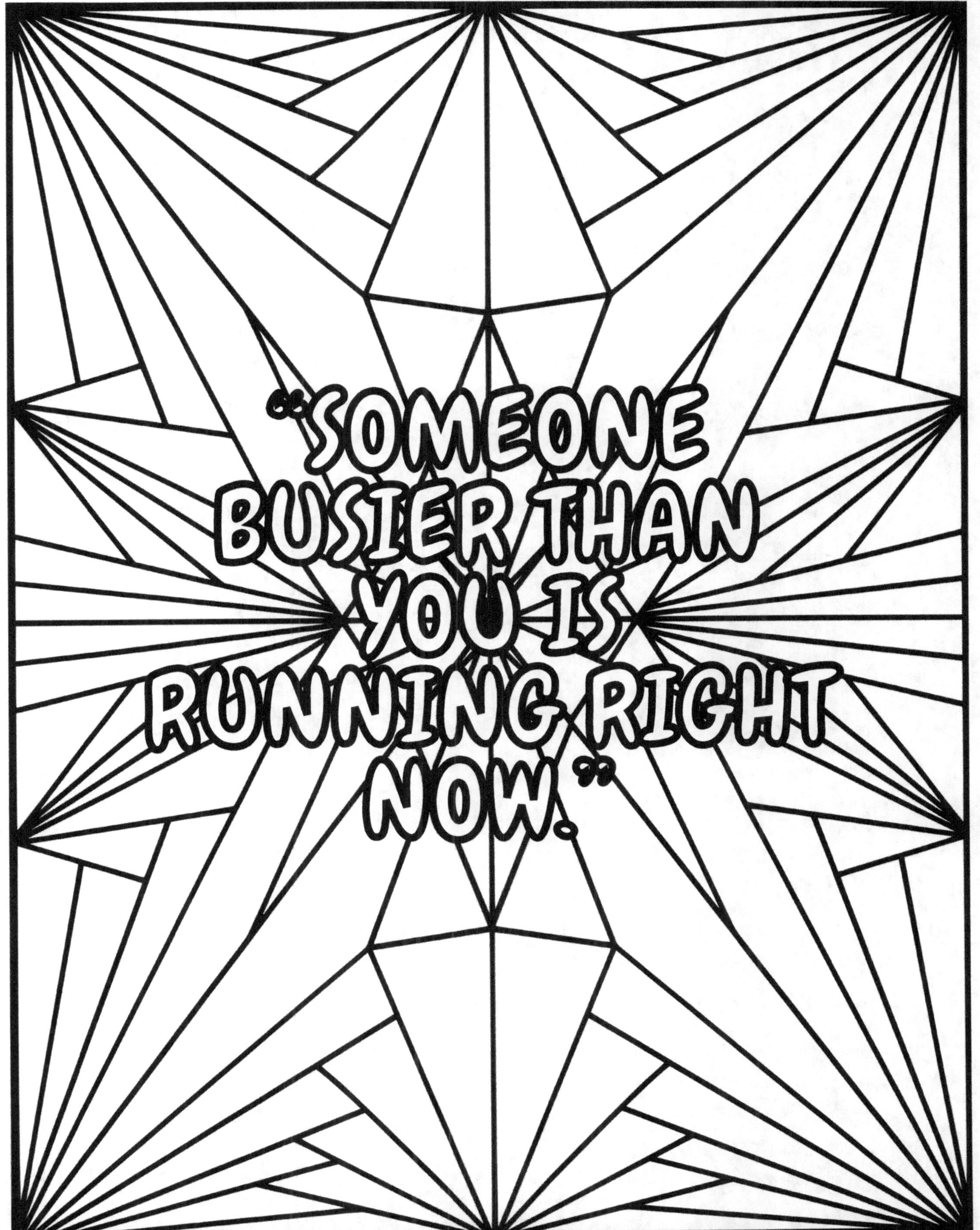

"SOMEONE BUSIER THAN YOU IS RUNNING RIGHT NOW."

"Someone busier than you is running right now."

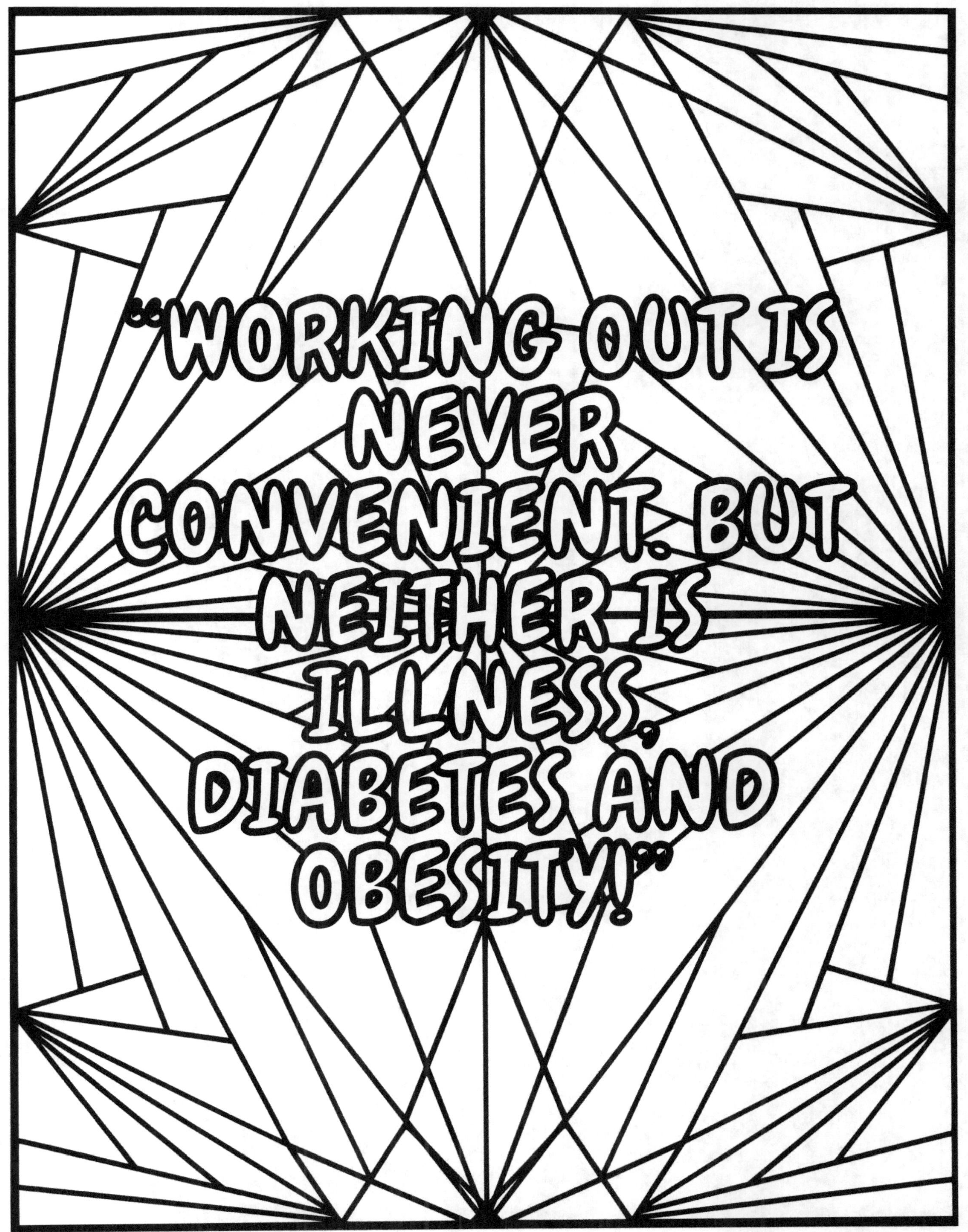

"WORKING OUT IS NEVER CONVENIENT. BUT NEITHER IS ILLNESS, DIABETES AND OBESITY!"

"Working out is never convenient. But neither is illness, diabetes and obesity!"

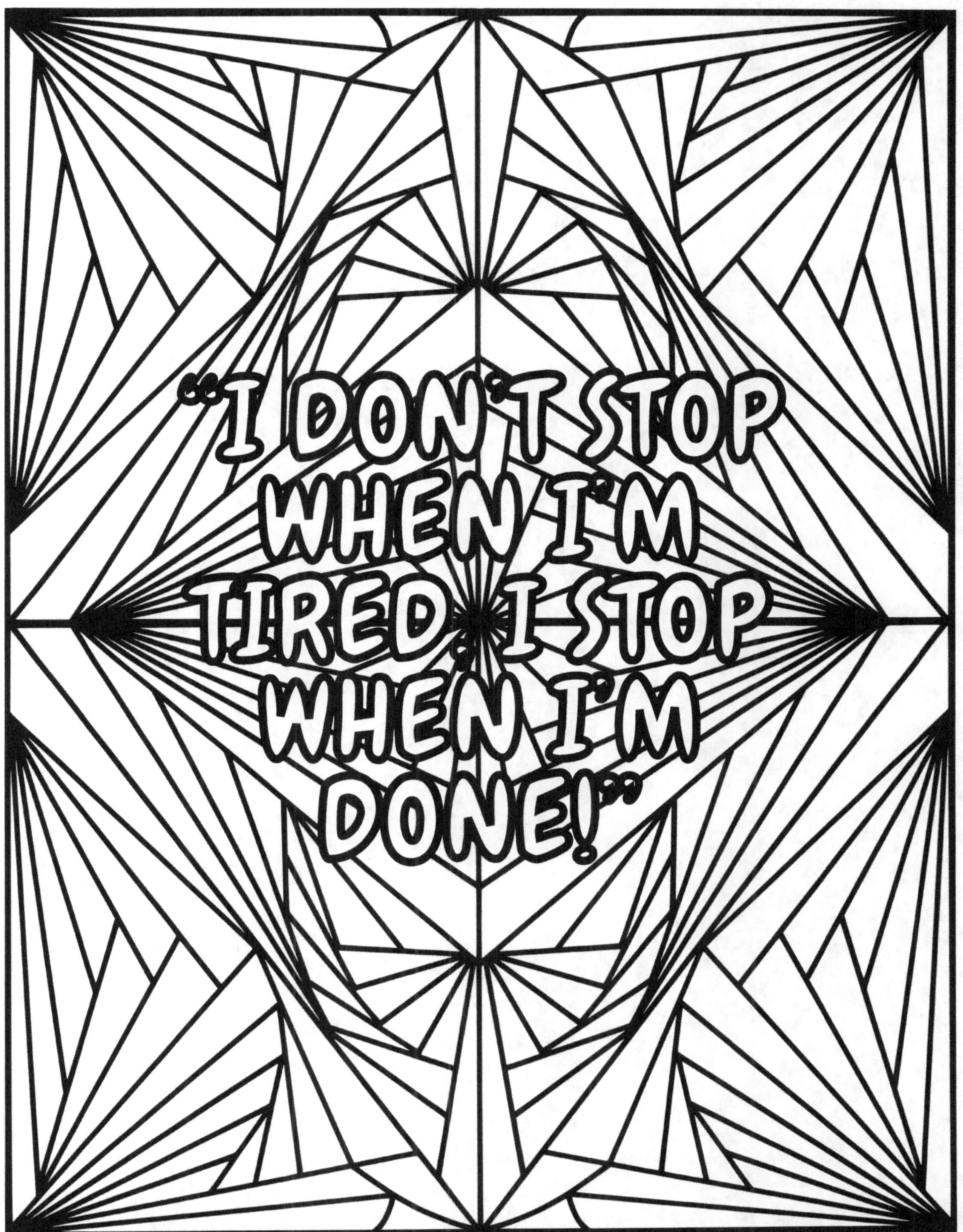

"I DON'T STOP WHEN I'M TIRED. I STOP WHEN I'M DONE!"

"I don't stop when I'm tired,
I stop when I'm DONE!"

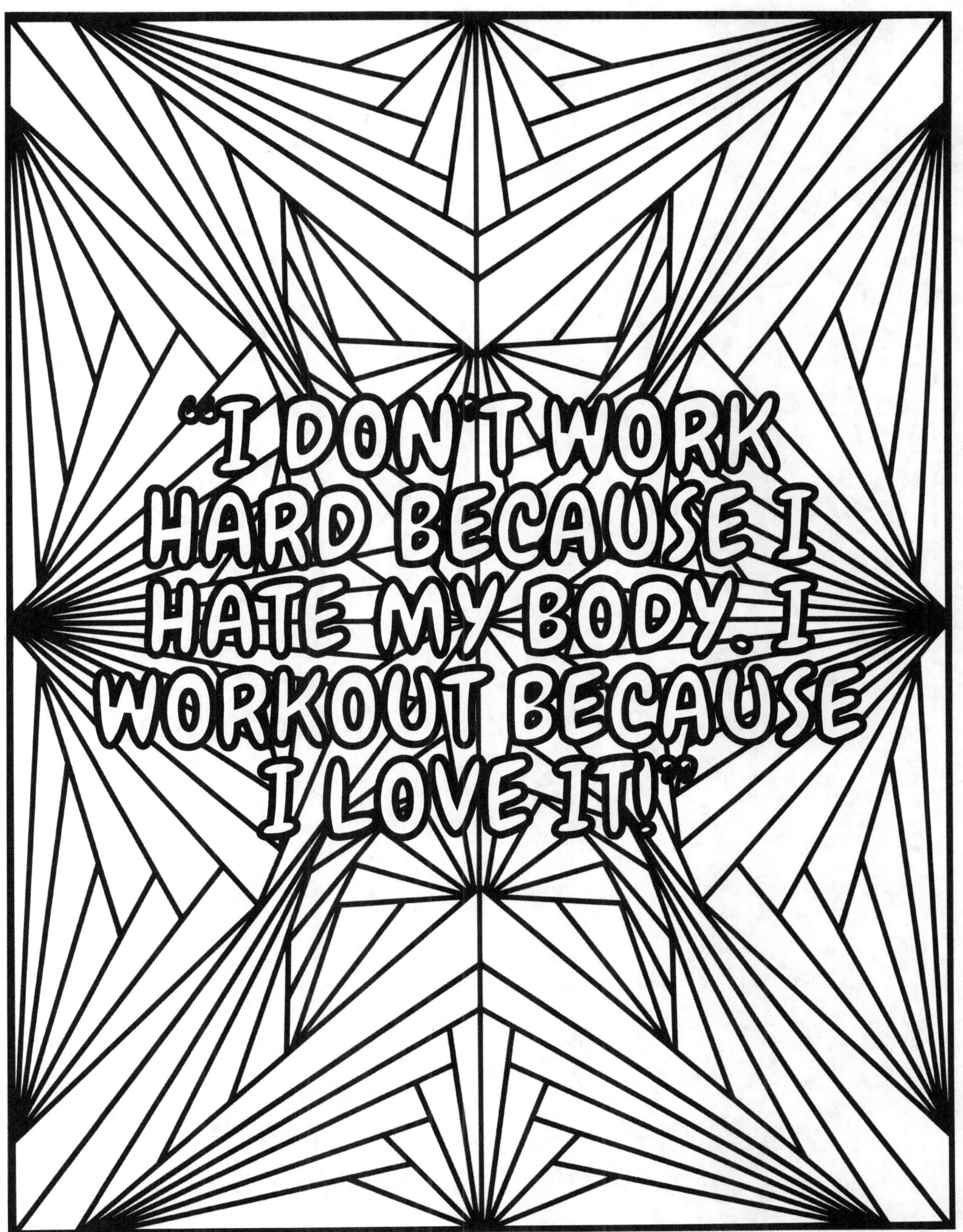
"I DON'T WORK HARD BECAUSE I HATE MY BODY. I WORKOUT BECAUSE I LOVE IT!"

"I don't work hard because I hate my body.
I workout because I love it!"

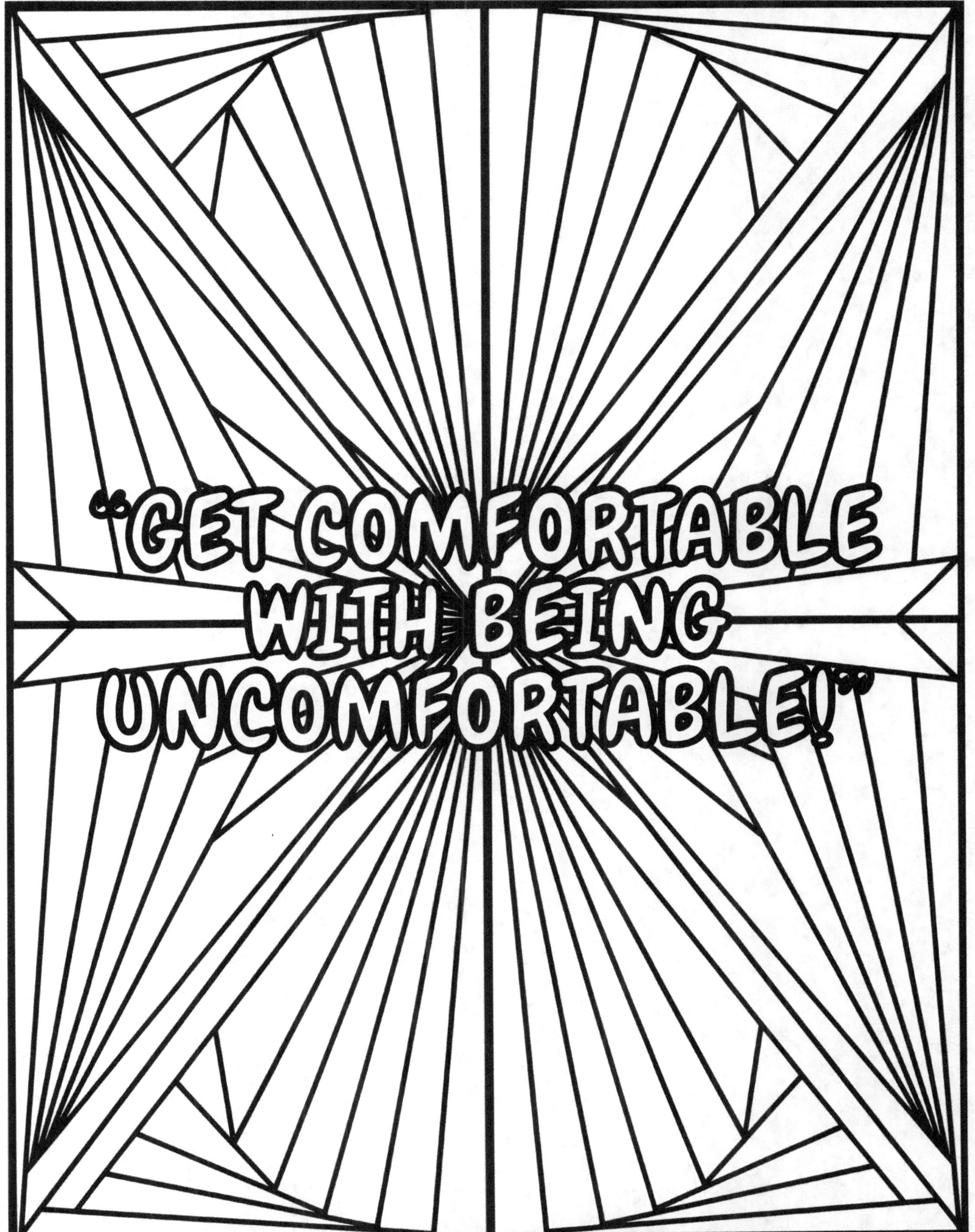

"GET COMFORTABLE WITH BEING UNCOMFORTABLE!"

"Get comfortable with being uncomfortable!"

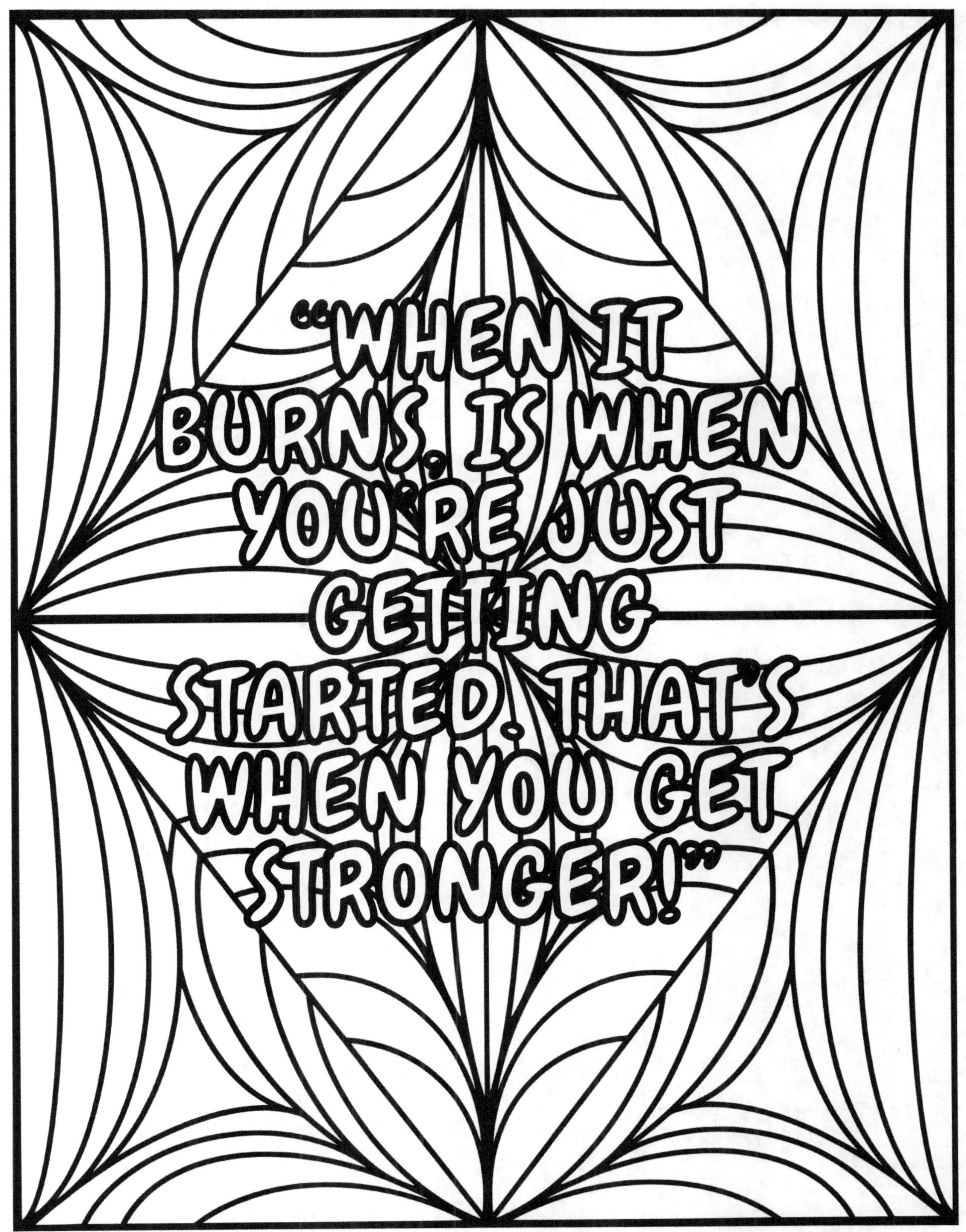
"WHEN IT BURNS, IS WHEN YOU'RE JUST GETTING STARTED. THAT'S WHEN YOU GET STRONGER!"

"When it burns, is when you're just getting started. That's when you get stronger!"

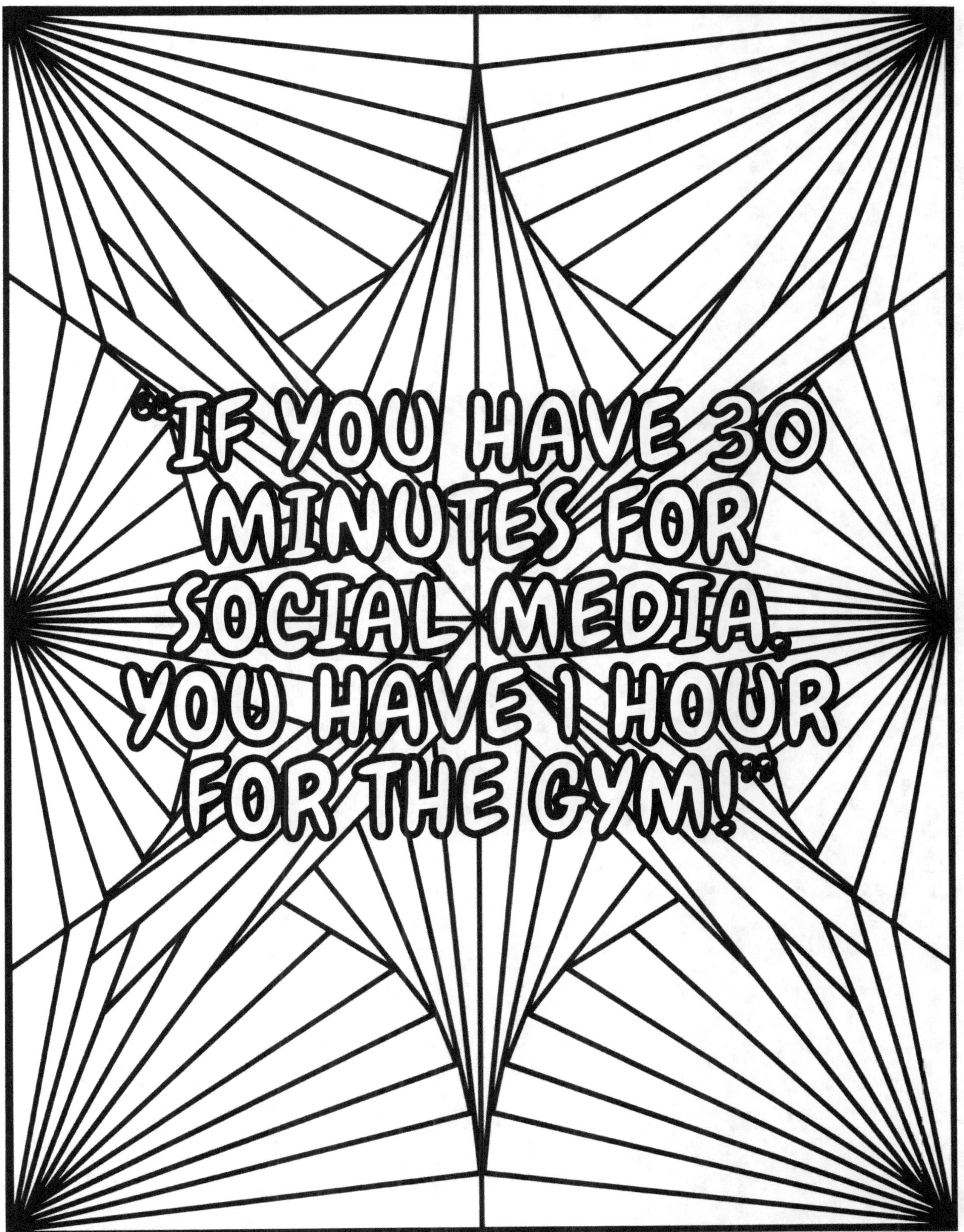
"IF YOU HAVE 30 MINUTES FOR SOCIAL MEDIA, YOU HAVE 1 HOUR FOR THE GYM!"

" If you have 30 minutes for social media,
you have 1 hour for the gym!"

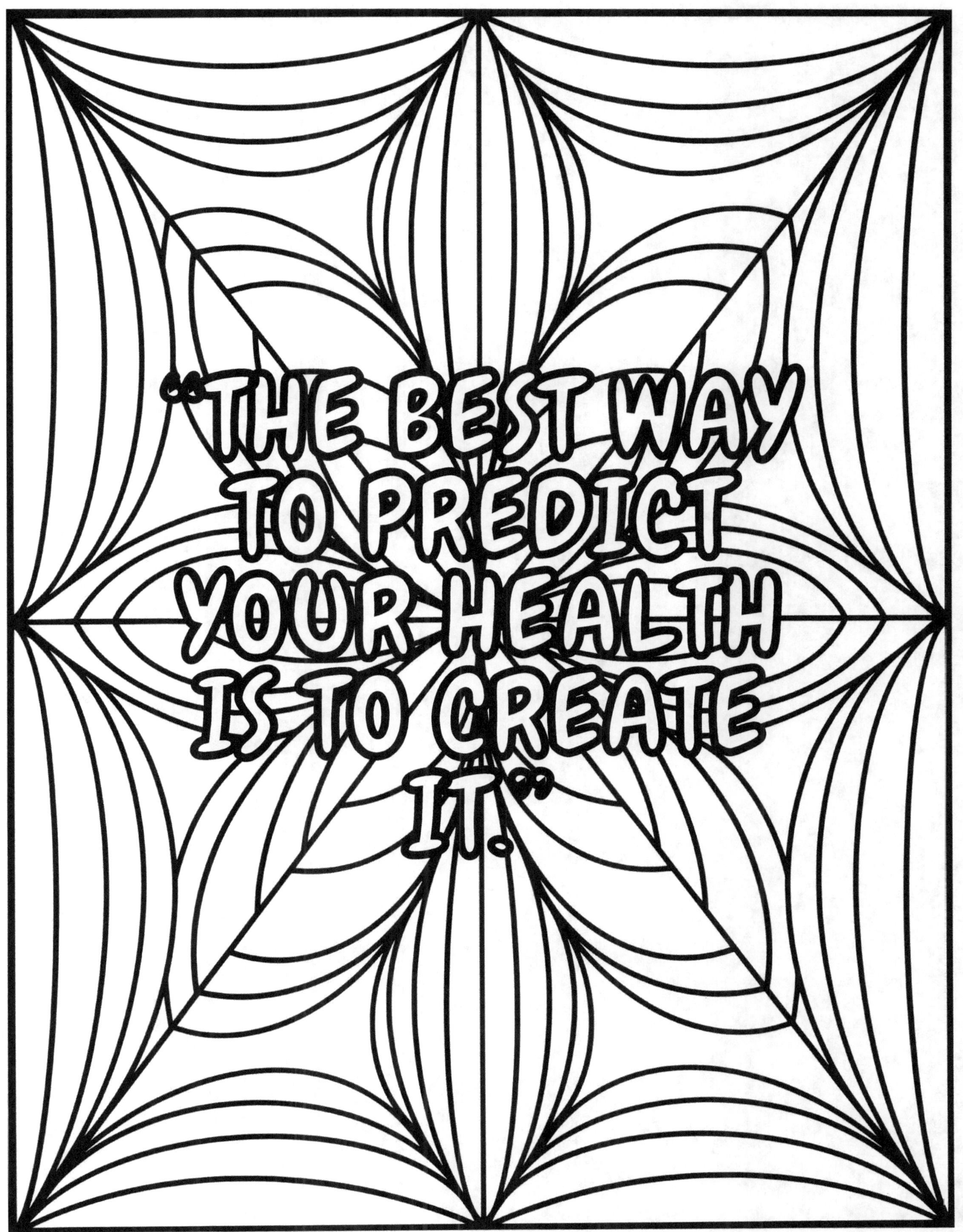
"THE BEST WAY TO PREDICT YOUR HEALTH IS TO CREATE IT."

"The best way to predict your health is to create it."

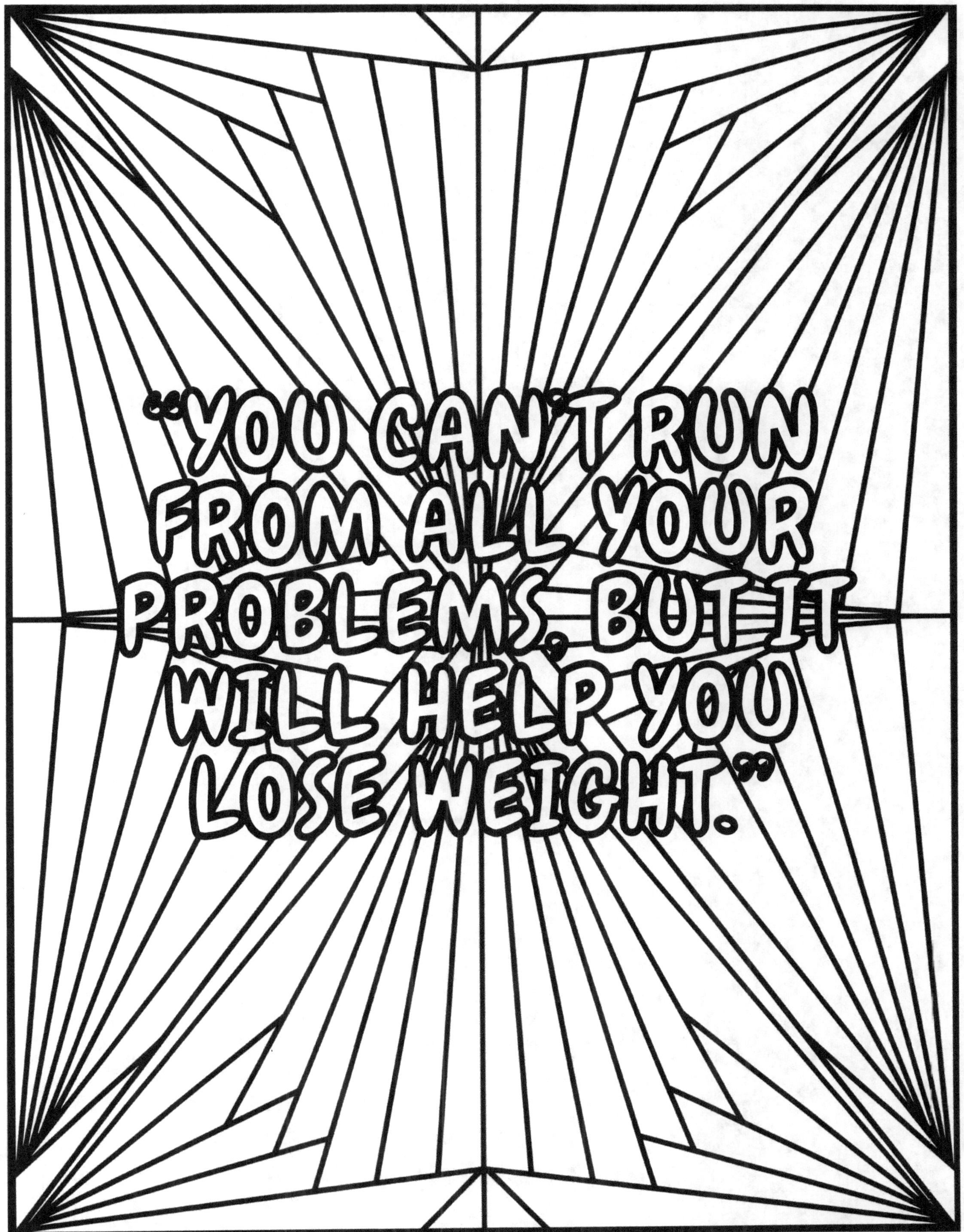

"YOU CAN'T RUN FROM ALL YOUR PROBLEMS, BUT IT WILL HELP YOU LOSE WEIGHT."

"You can't run from all your problems,
but it will help you lose weight."

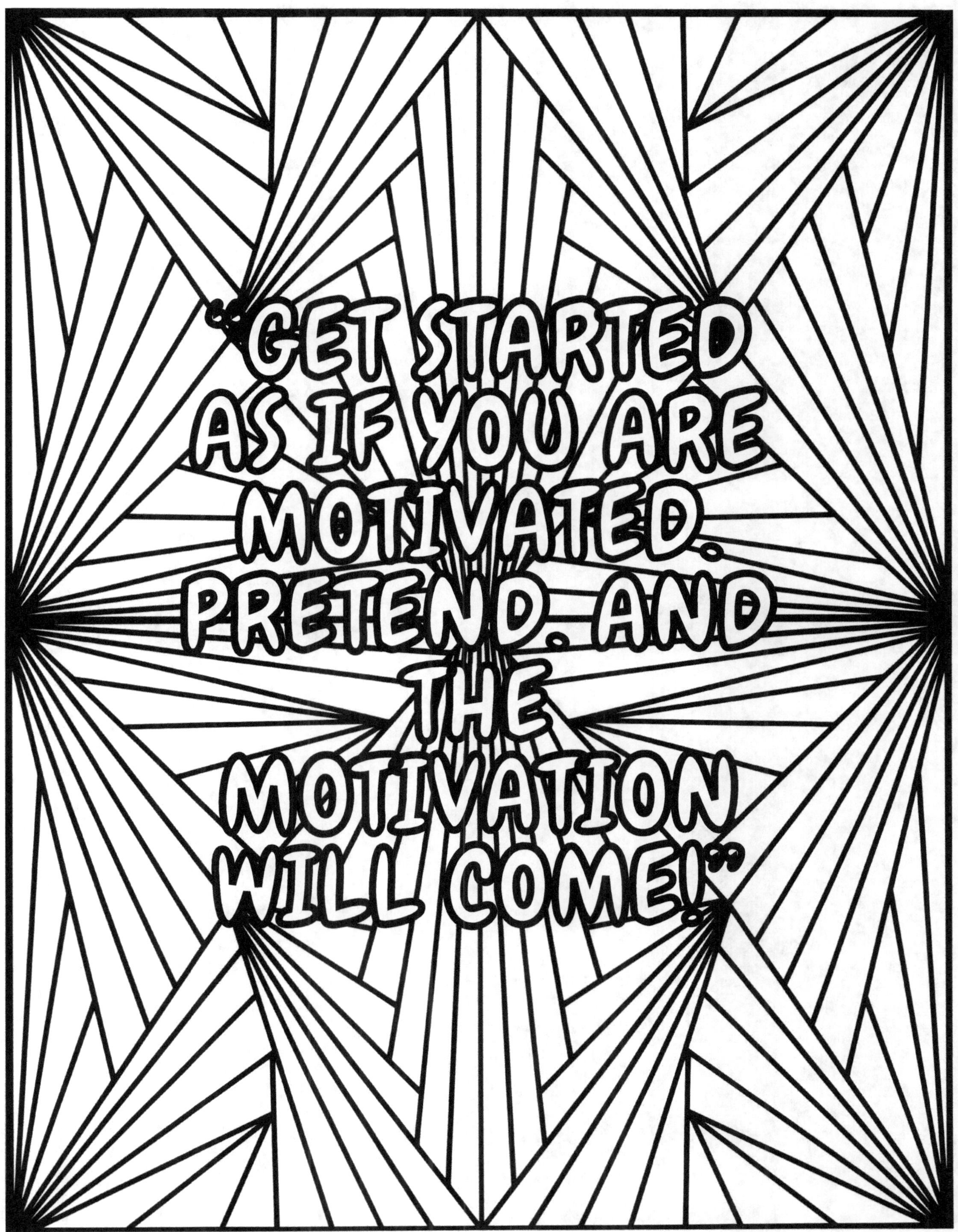

"GET STARTED AS IF YOU ARE MOTIVATED. PRETEND. AND THE MOTIVATION WILL COME!"

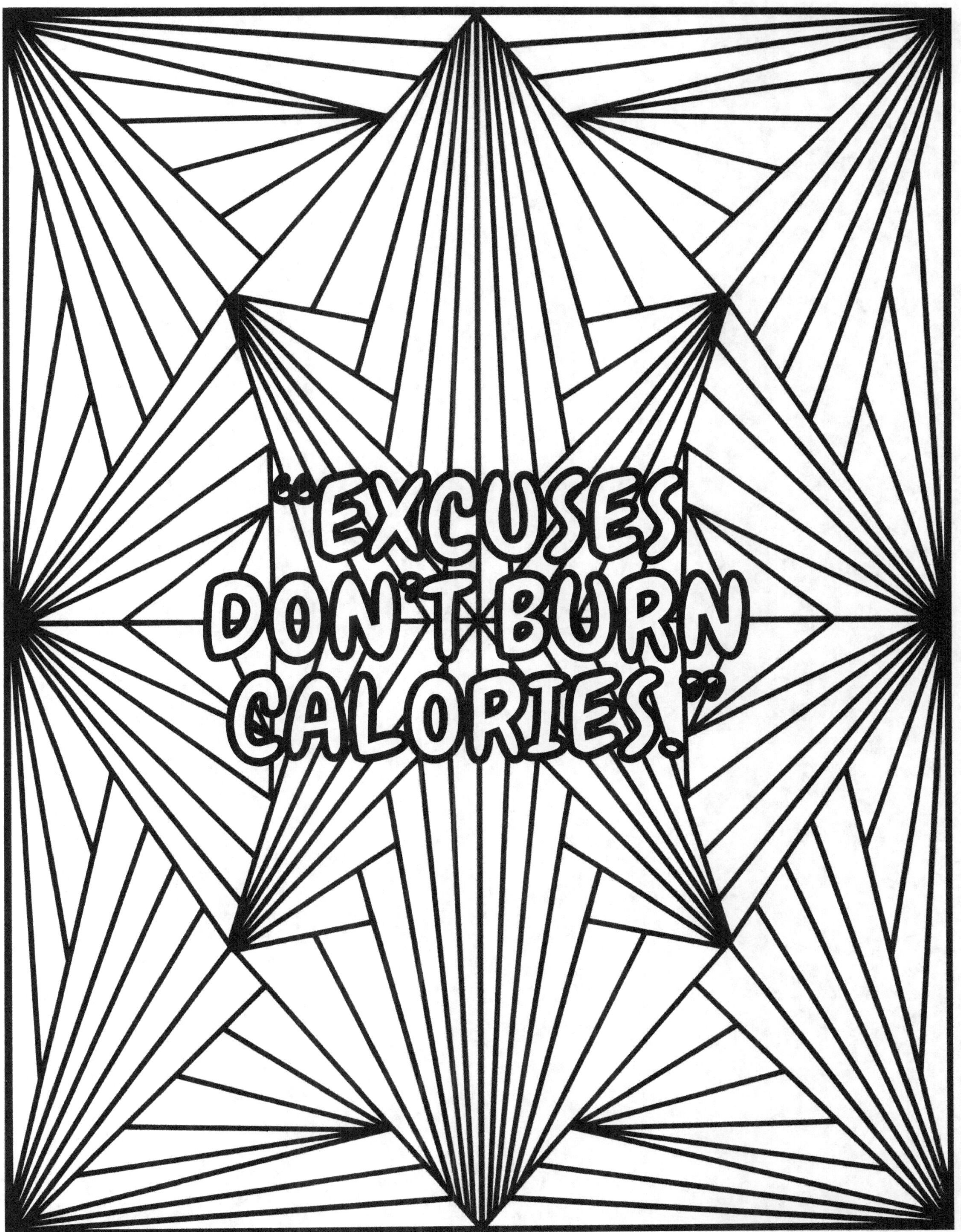

"EXCUSES DON'T BURN CALORIES."

"Excuses don't burn calories."

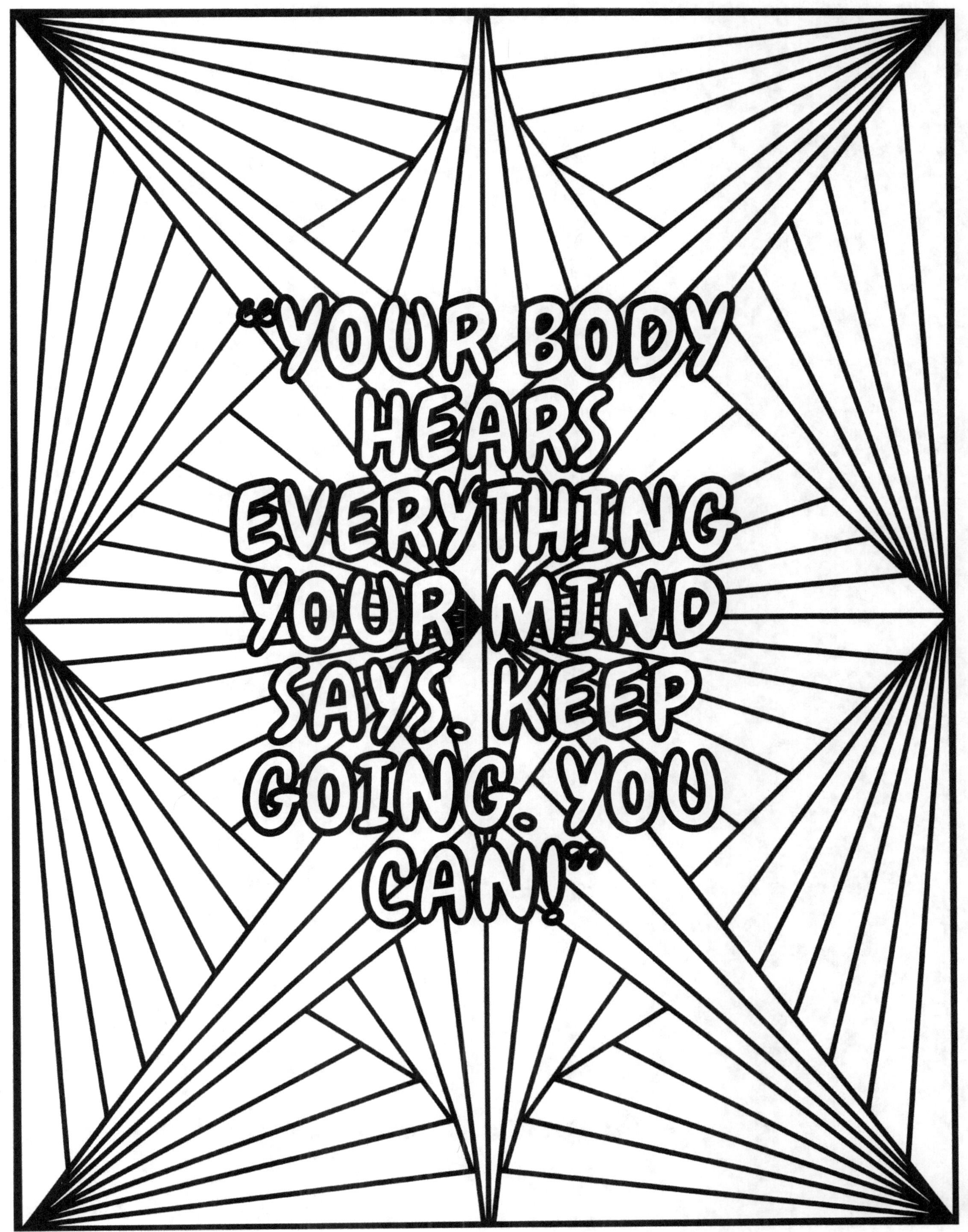

"YOUR BODY HEARS EVERYTHING YOUR MIND SAYS. KEEP GOING. YOU CAN!"

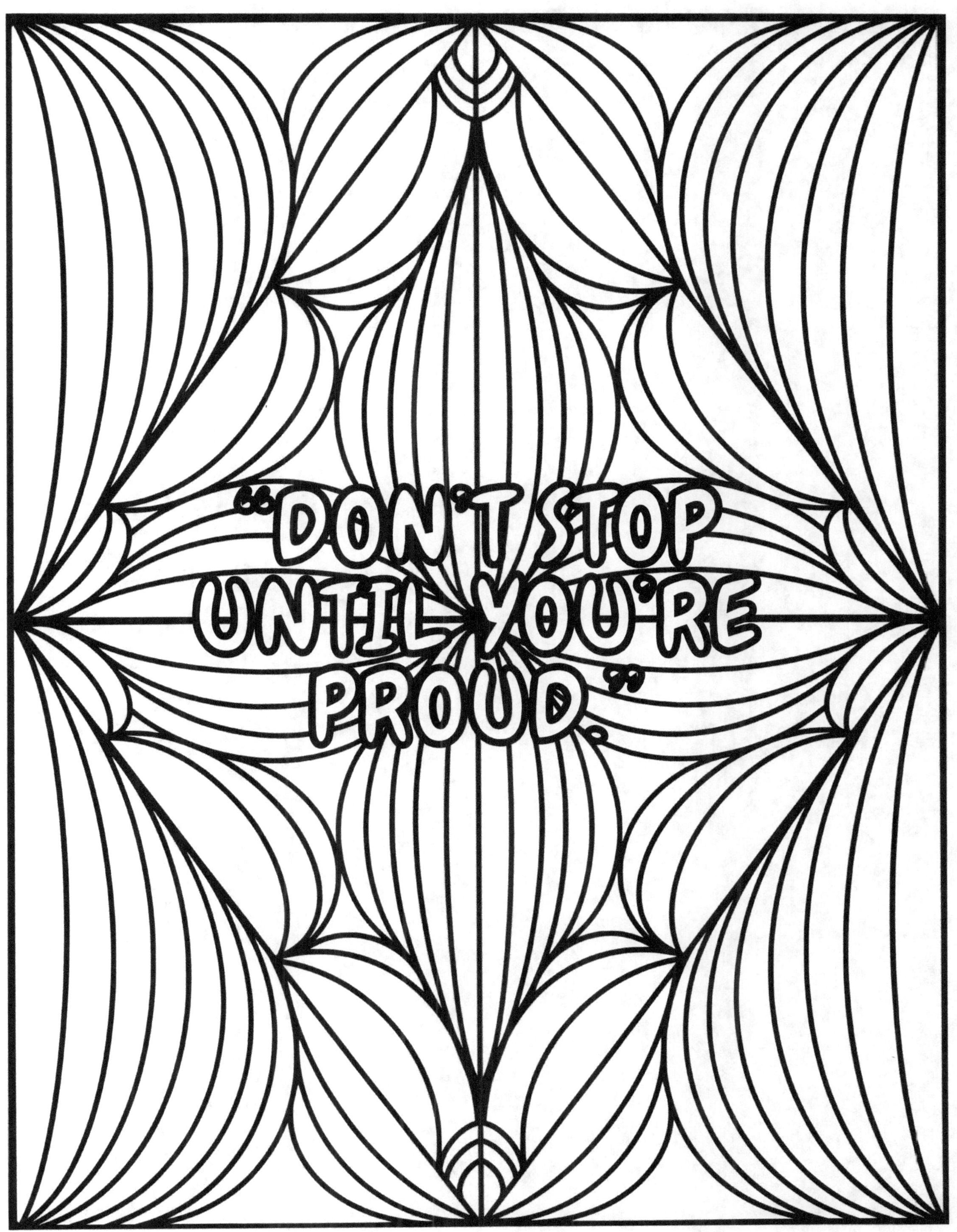

"DON'T STOP UNTIL YOU'RE PROUD."

"Don't stop until you're proud."

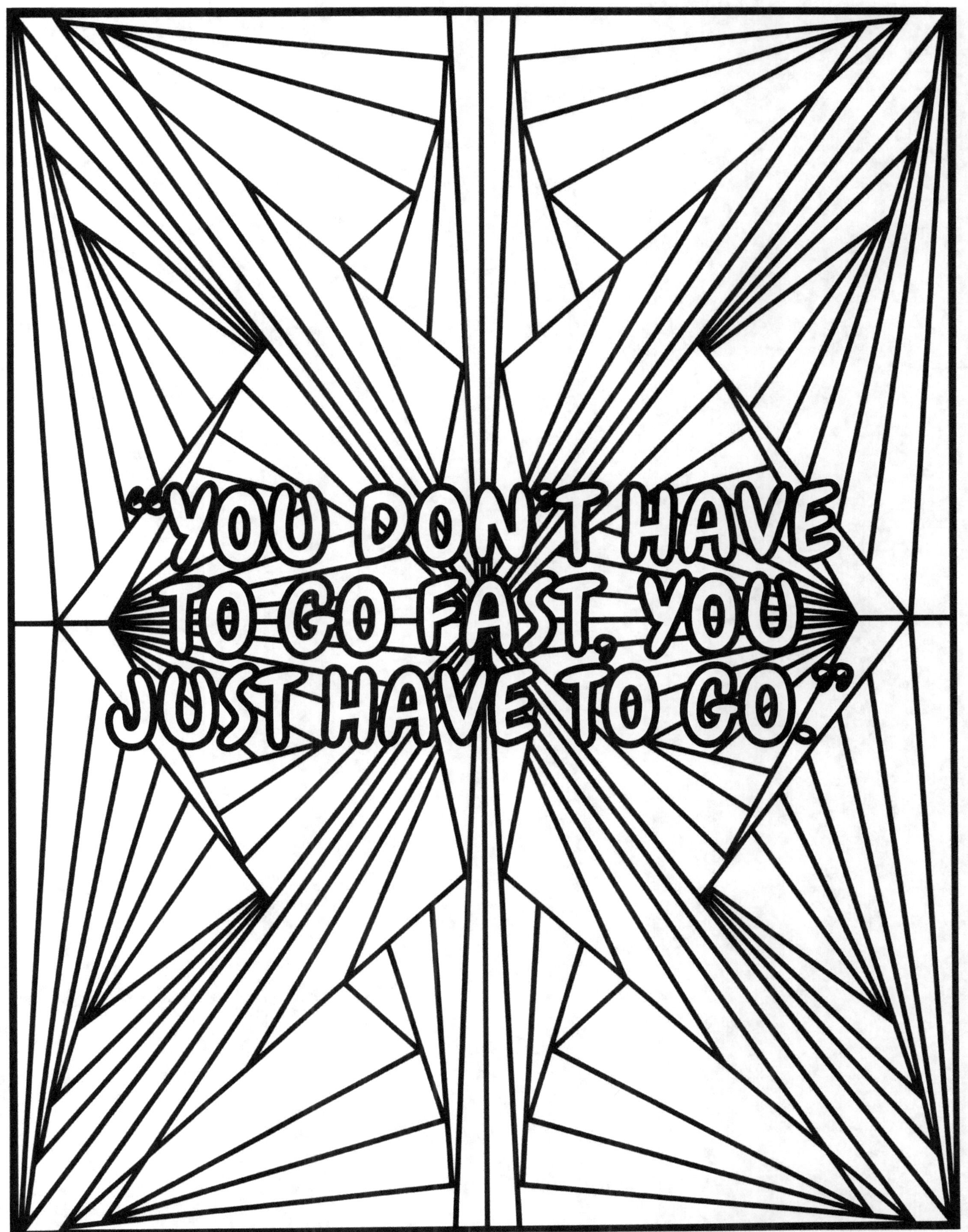

"YOU DON'T HAVE TO GO FAST, YOU JUST HAVE TO GO."

"You don't have to go fast,
you just have to go."

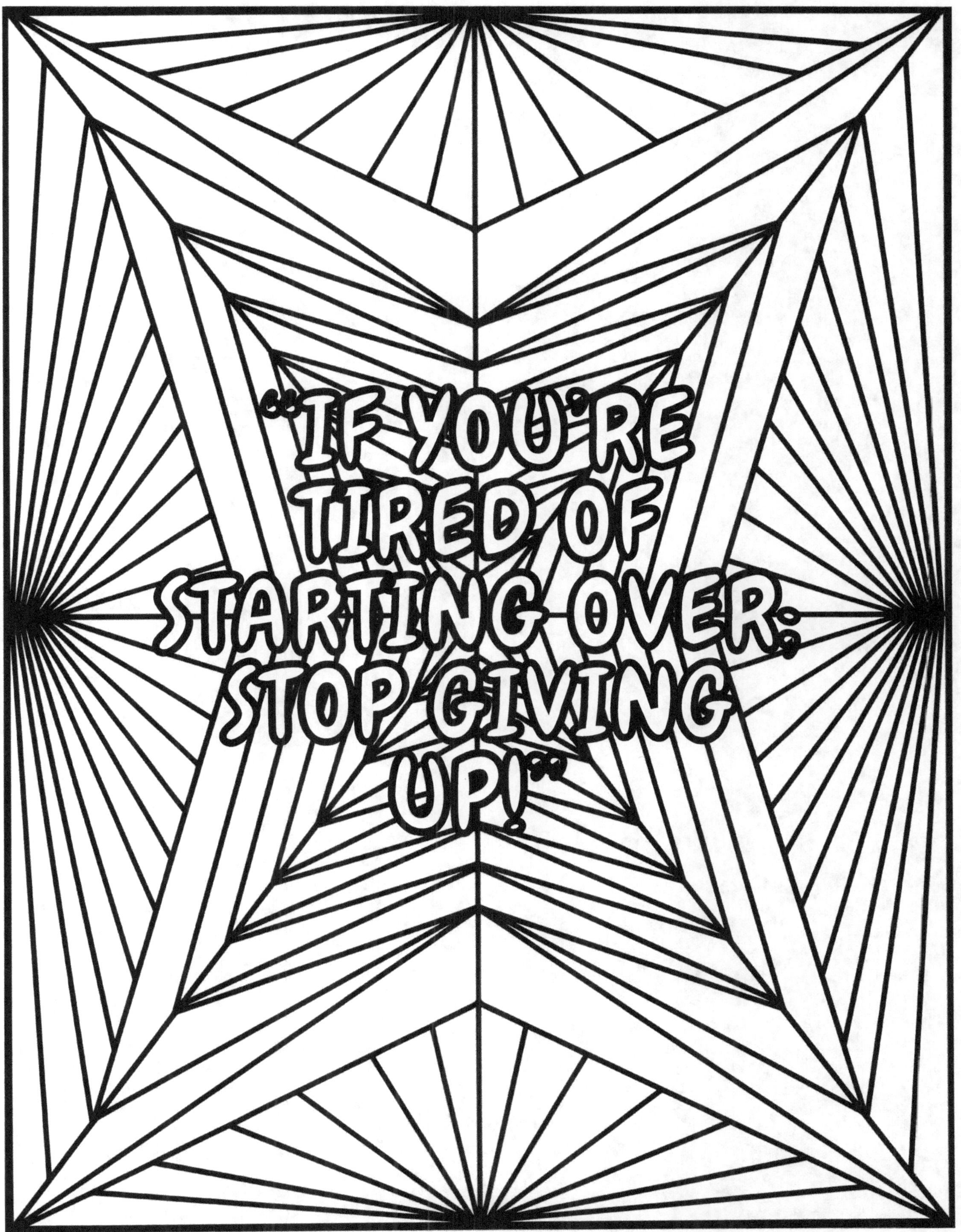

"IF YOU'RE
TIRED OF
STARTING OVER,
STOP GIVING
UP!"

"If you're tired of starting over; stop giving up!"

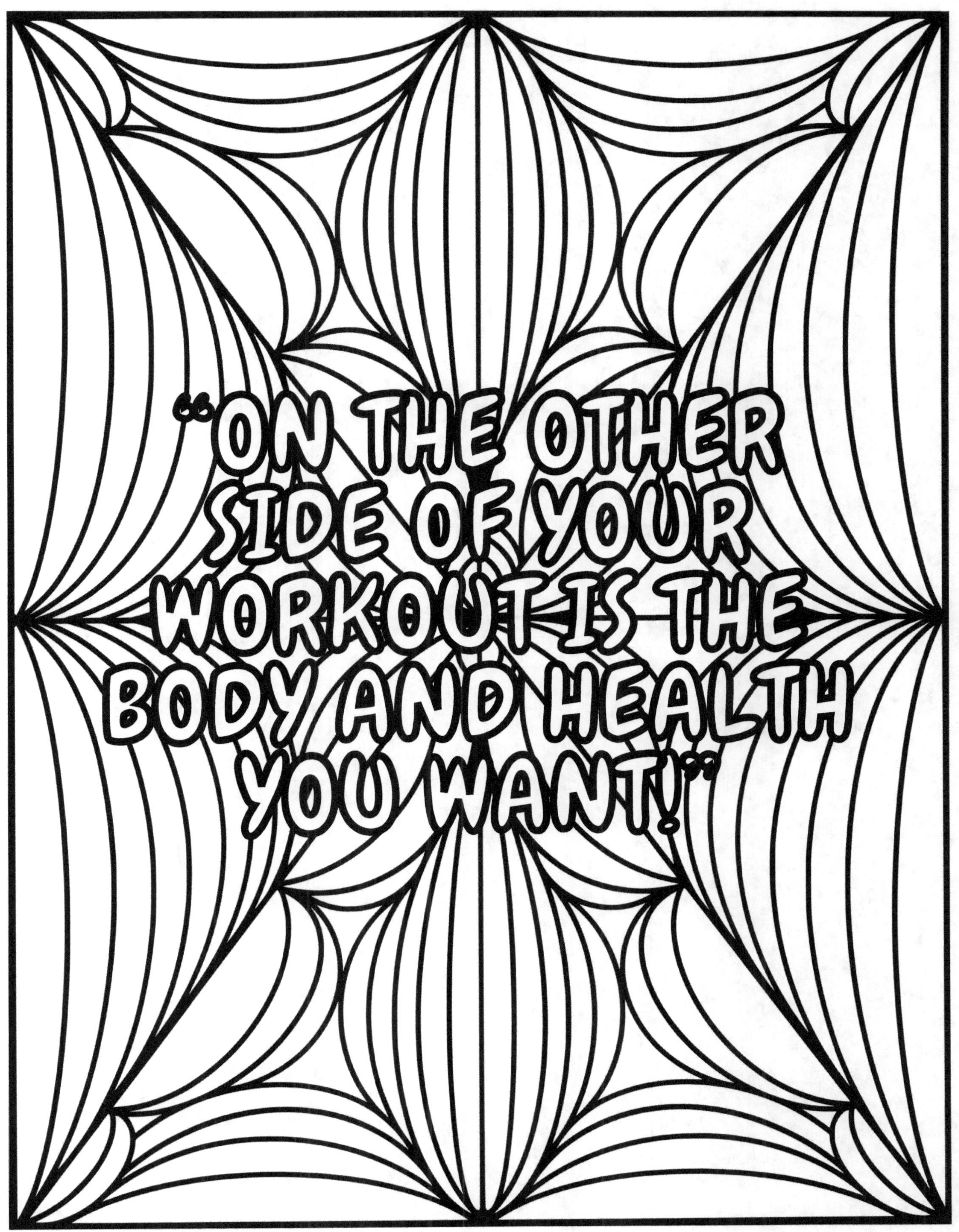

"ON THE OTHER SIDE OF YOUR WORKOUT IS THE BODY AND HEALTH YOU WANT!"

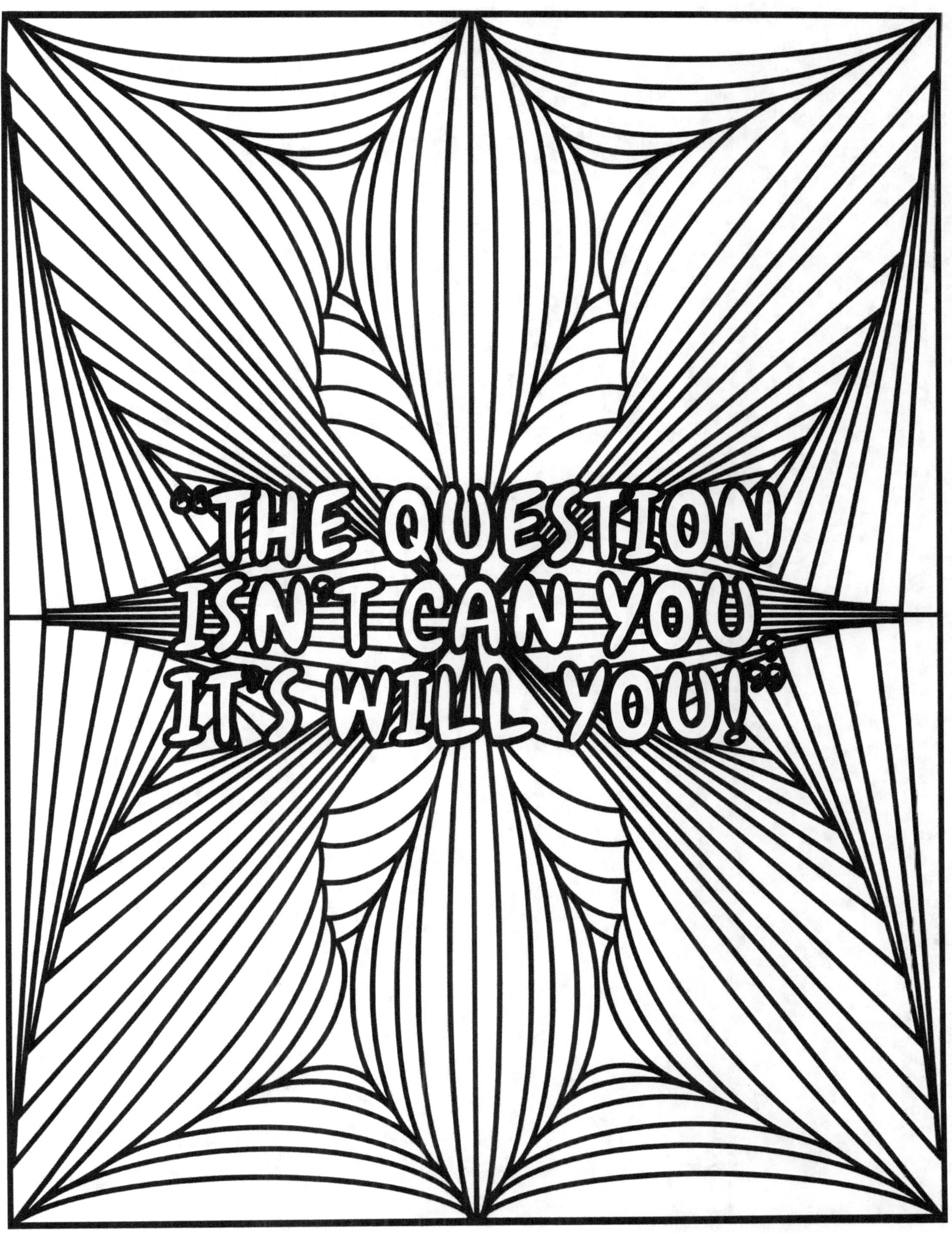

"THE QUESTION ISN'T CAN YOU. IT'S WILL YOU!"

"The question isn't can you, it's will you!"

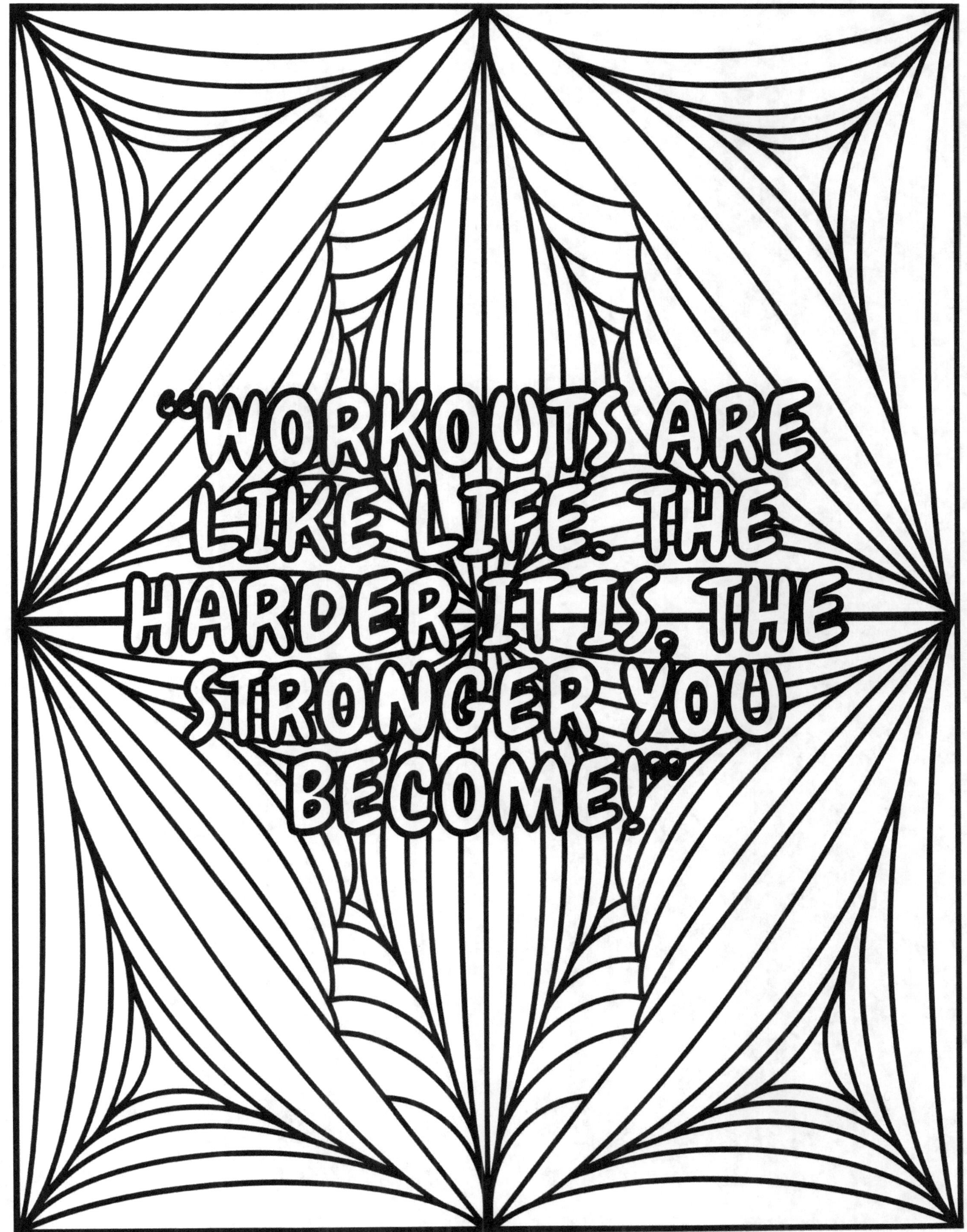

"WORKOUTS ARE LIKE LIFE. THE HARDER IT IS, THE STRONGER YOU BECOME!"

"Workouts are like life. The harder it is, the STRONGER YOU BECOME!"

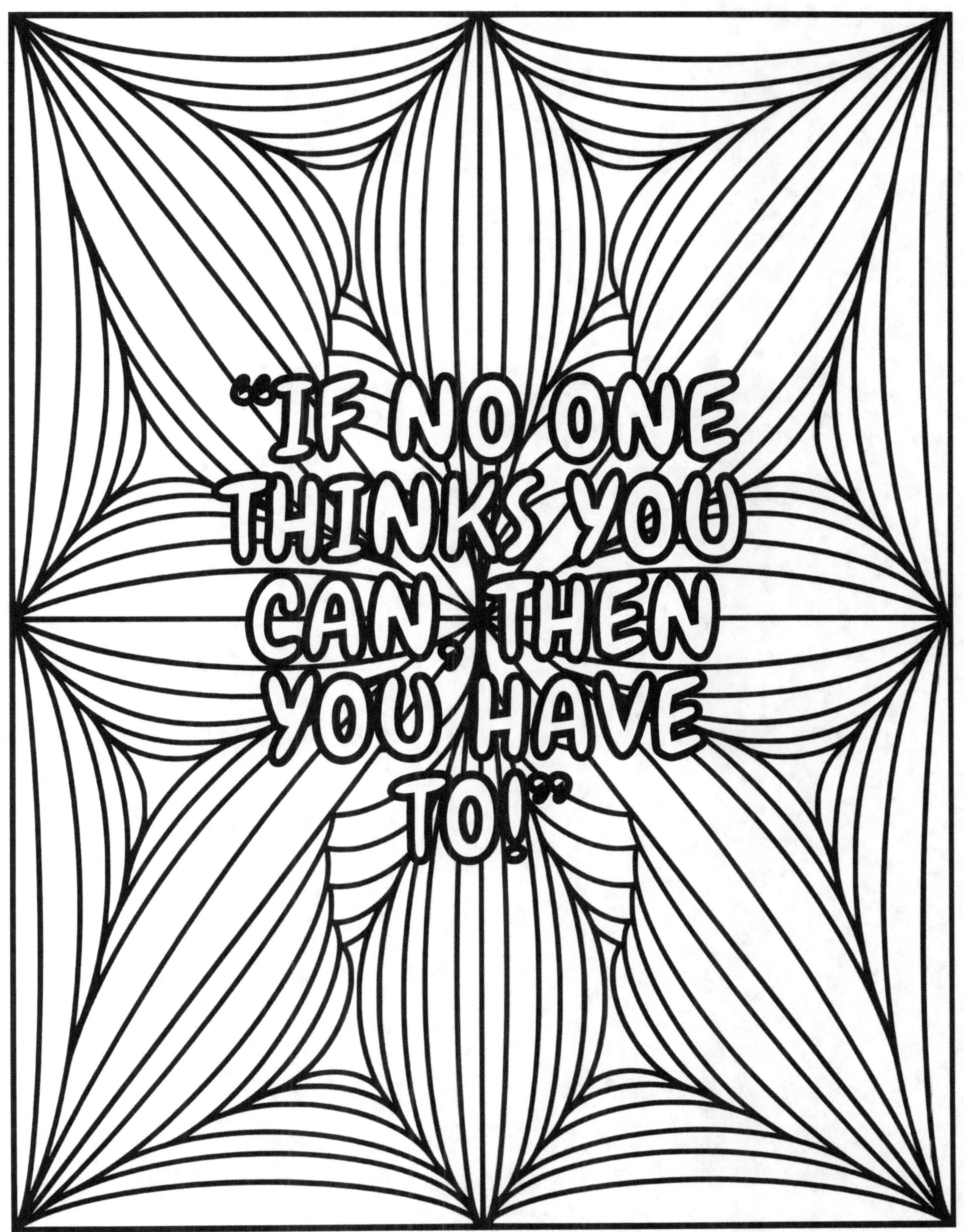

"IF NO ONE THINKS YOU CAN, THEN YOU HAVE TO!"

"If no one thinks you can, then you have to!"

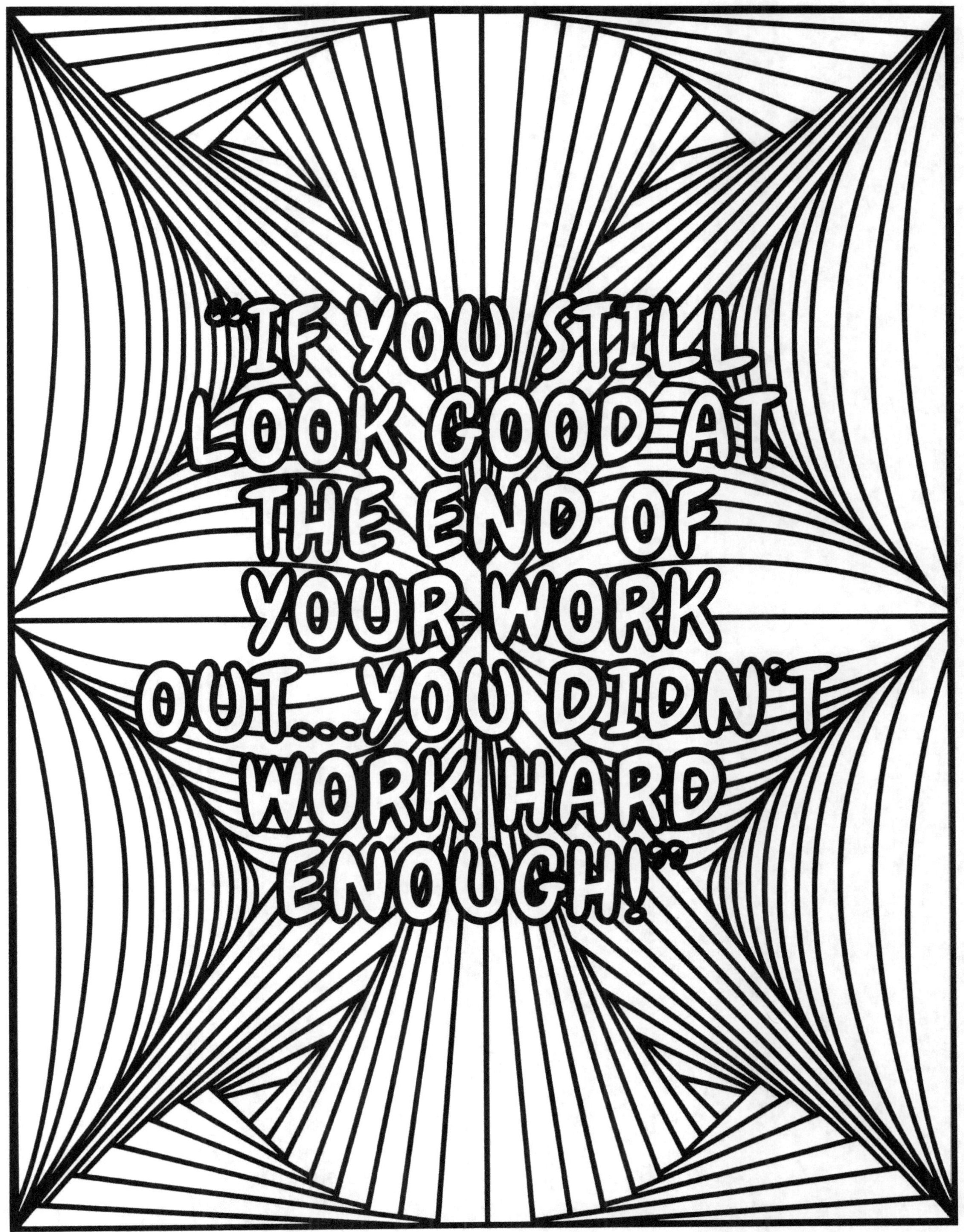

"IF YOU STILL LOOK GOOD AT THE END OF YOUR WORK OUT.... YOU DIDN'T WORK HARD ENOUGH!"

" If you still look good at the end of your work out...you didn't work hard enough!"

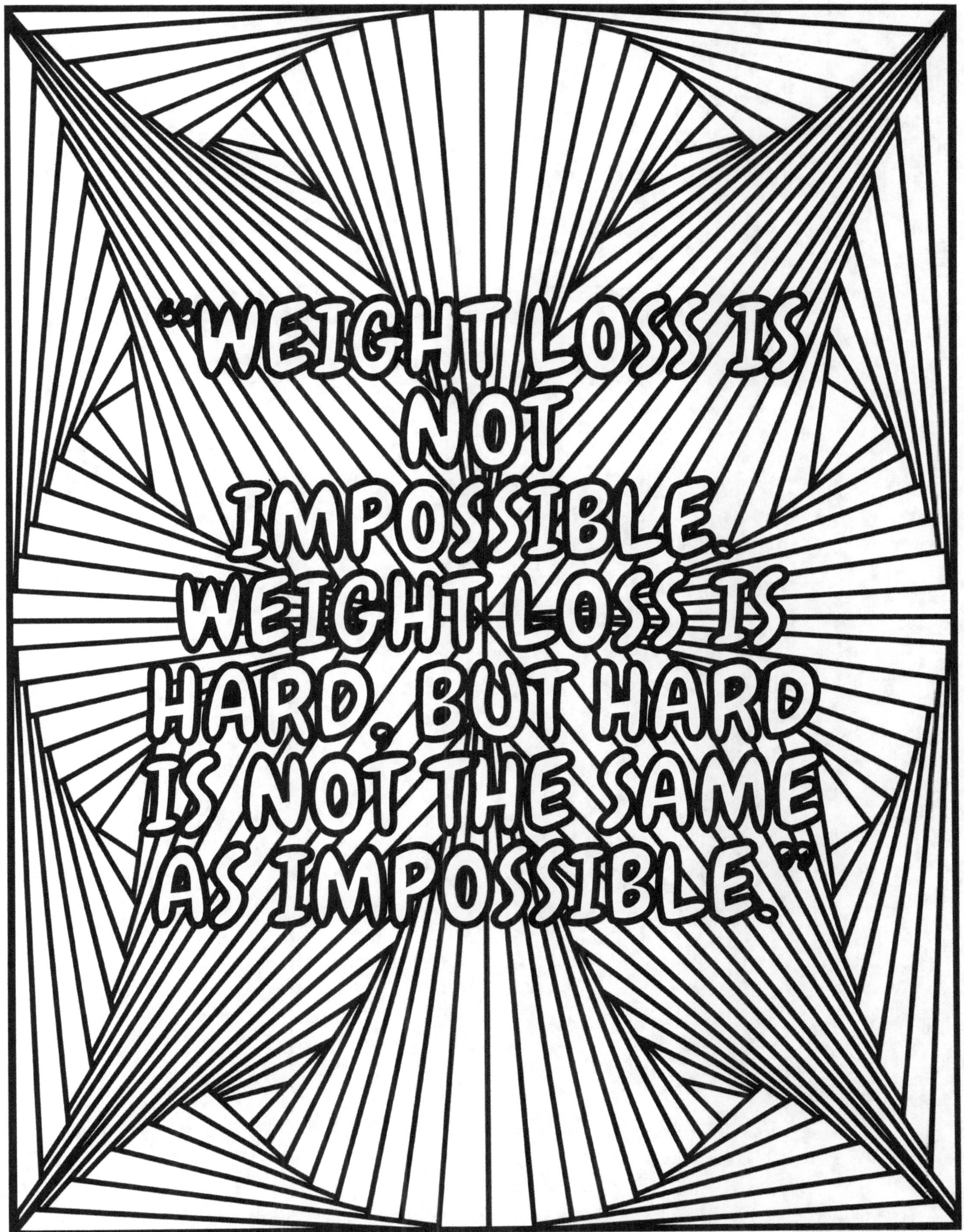
"WEIGHT LOSS IS NOT IMPOSSIBLE. WEIGHT LOSS IS HARD. BUT HARD IS NOT THE SAME AS IMPOSSIBLE."

"Weight loss is not impossible. Weight loss is hard, but hard is not the same as impossible."

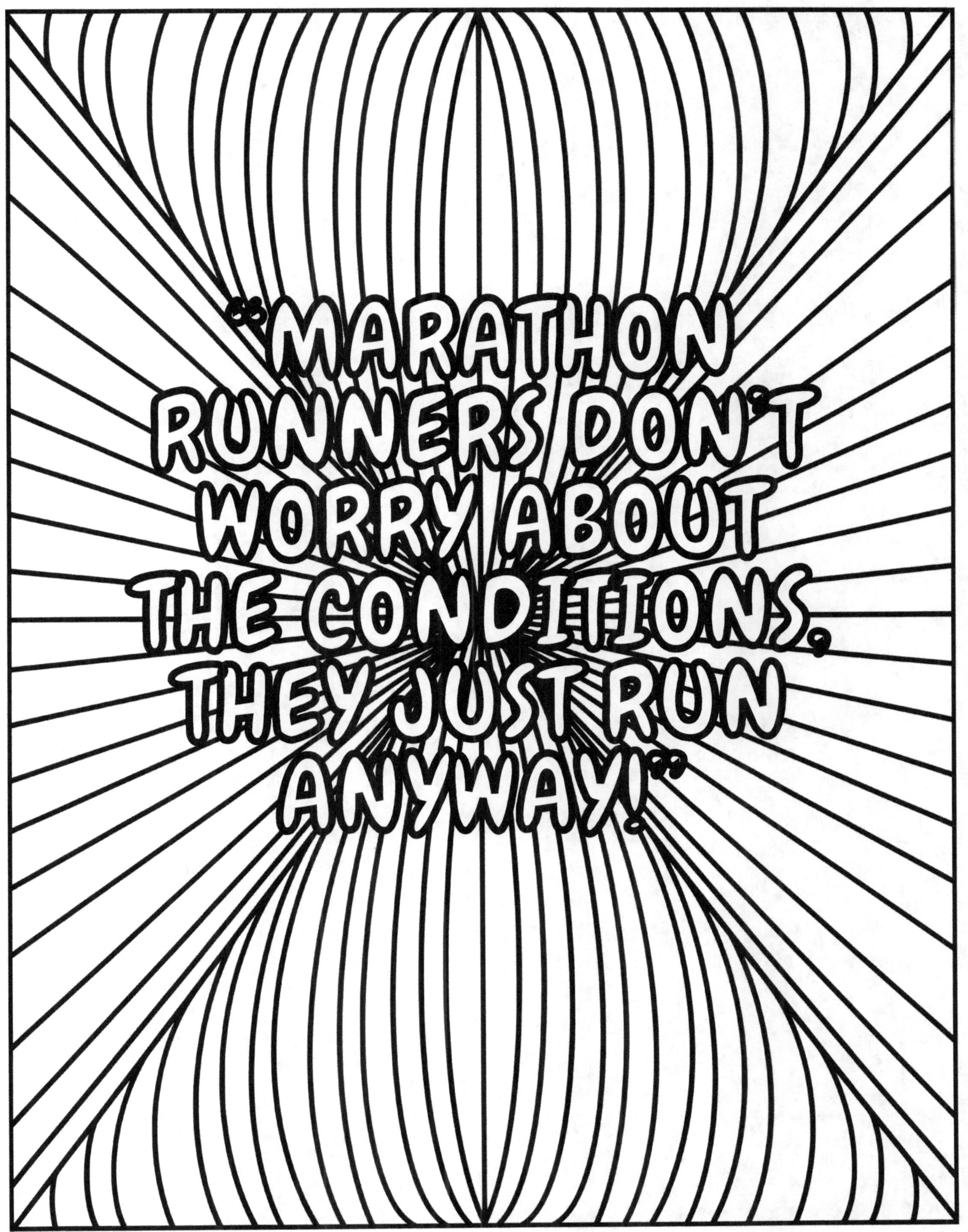

"MARATHON RUNNERS DON'T WORRY ABOUT THE CONDITIONS. THEY JUST RUN ANYWAY!"

"Marathon runners don't worry about the
conditions, they just run anyway!"

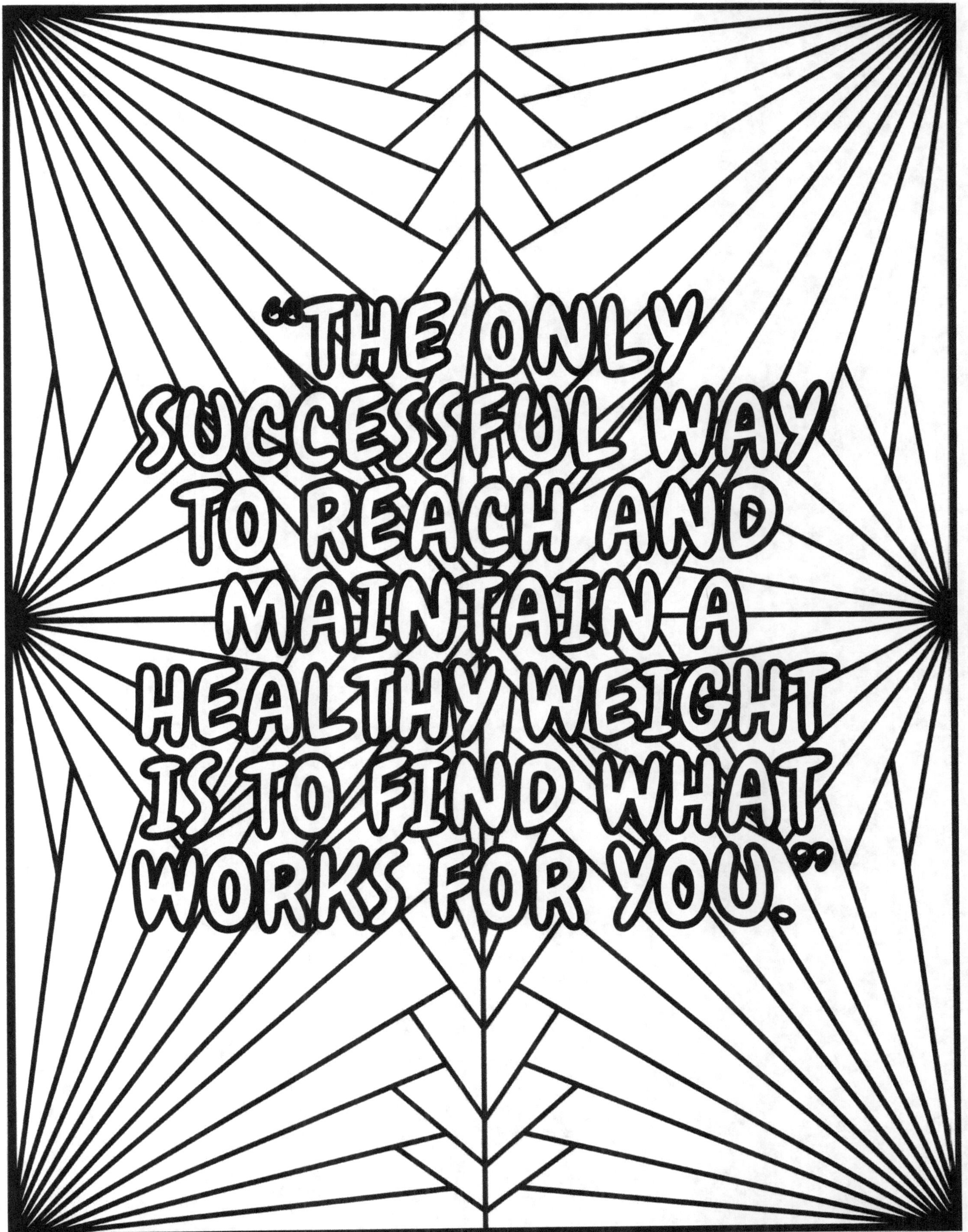

"THE ONLY SUCCESSFUL WAY TO REACH AND MAINTAIN A HEALTHY WEIGHT IS TO FIND WHAT WORKS FOR YOU."

"The only successful way to reach and maintain a healthy weight is to find what works for you."

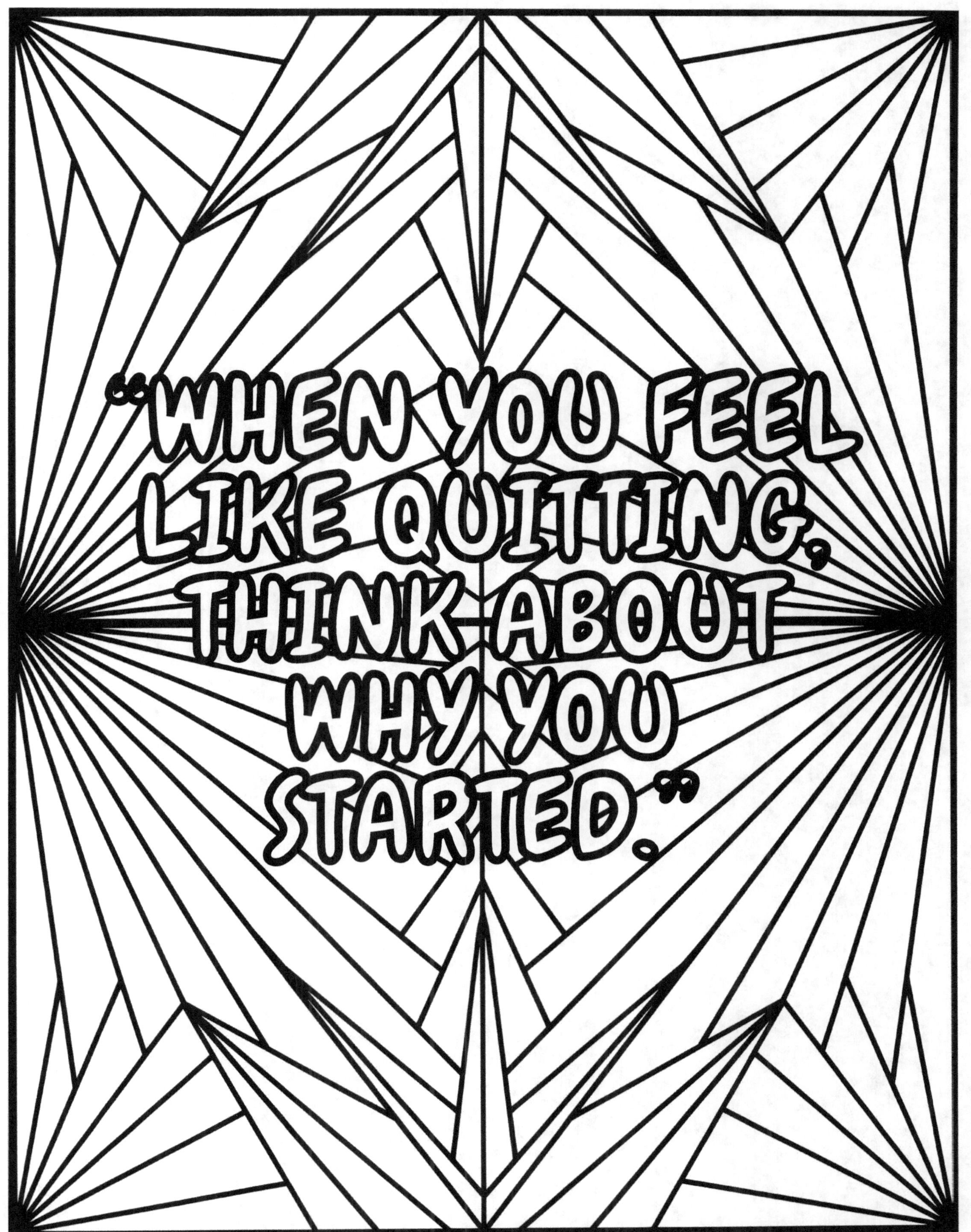
"WHEN YOU FEEL LIKE QUITTING, THINK ABOUT WHY YOU STARTED."

"When you feel like quitting, think about why you started."

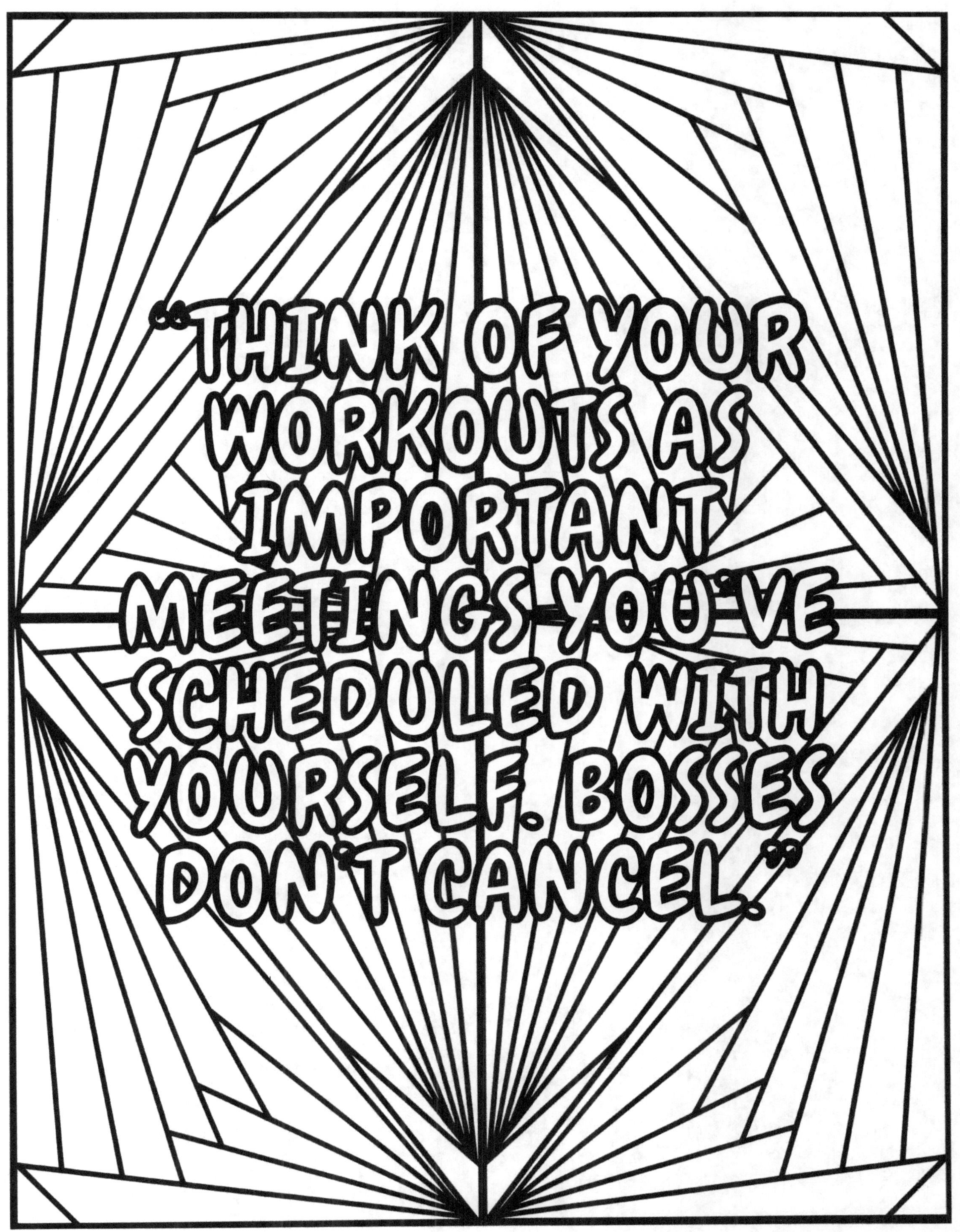
"THINK OF YOUR WORKOUTS AS IMPORTANT MEETINGS YOU'VE SCHEDULED WITH YOURSELF. BOSSES DON'T CANCEL."

"Think of your workouts as important meetings you've scheduled with yourself. Bosses don't cancel."

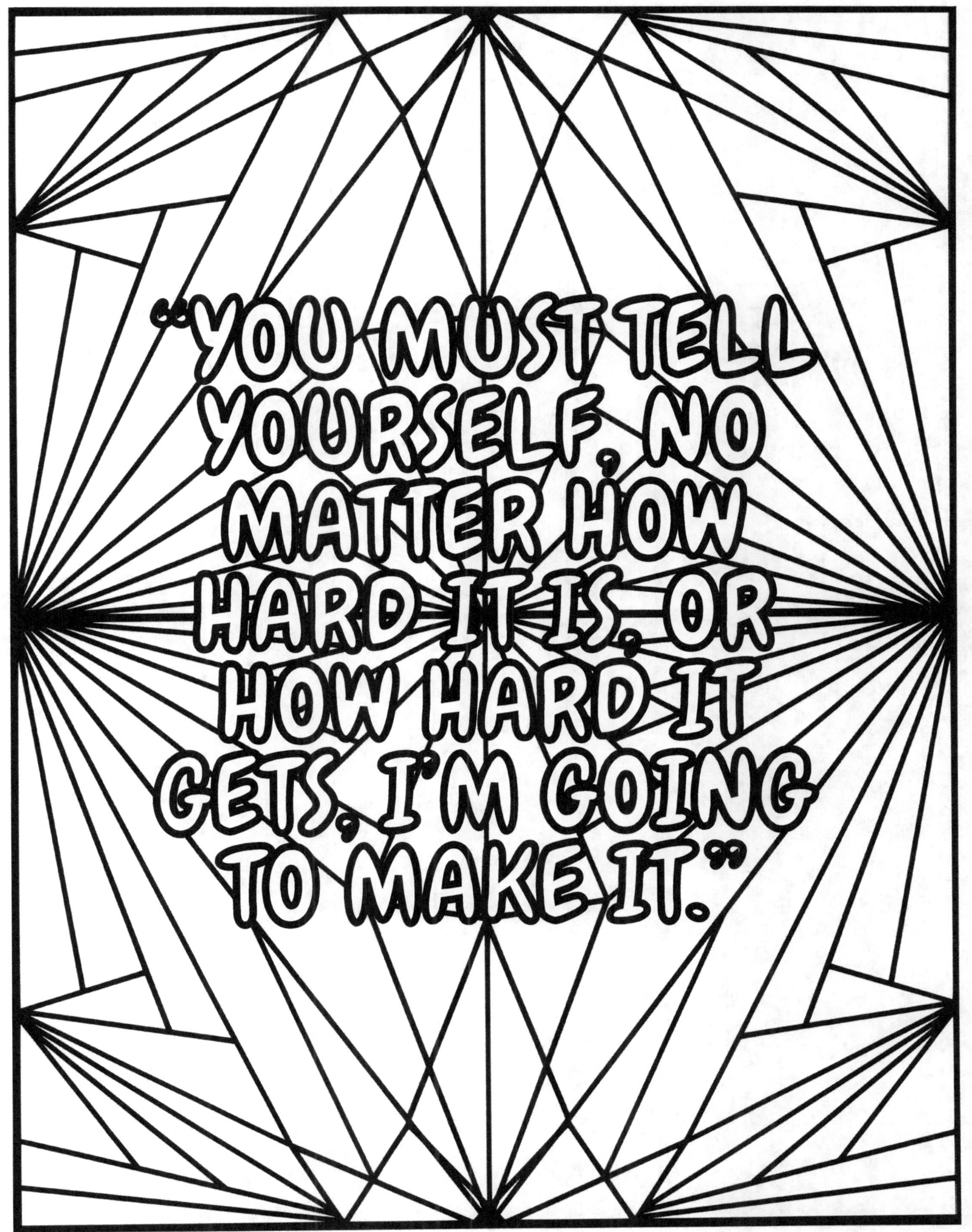

"YOU MUST TELL YOURSELF, NO MATTER HOW HARD IT IS, OR HOW HARD IT GETS, I'M GOING TO MAKE IT."

"You must tell yourself, no matter how hard it is, or how hard it gets, I'm going to make it."

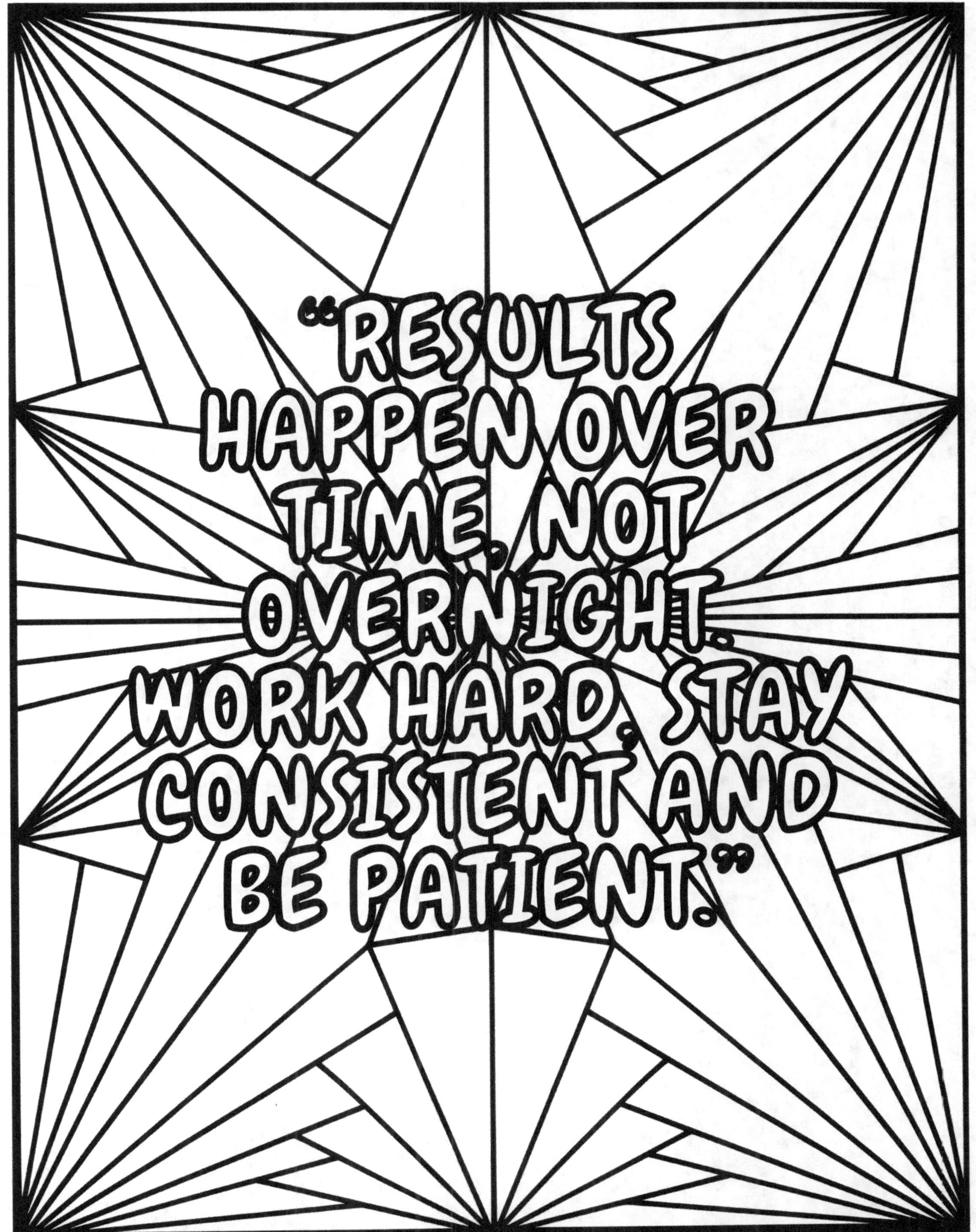

"RESULTS HAPPEN OVER TIME, NOT OVERNIGHT. WORK HARD, STAY CONSISTENT AND BE PATIENT."

"Results happen over time, not overnight. Work hard, stay consistent and be patient."

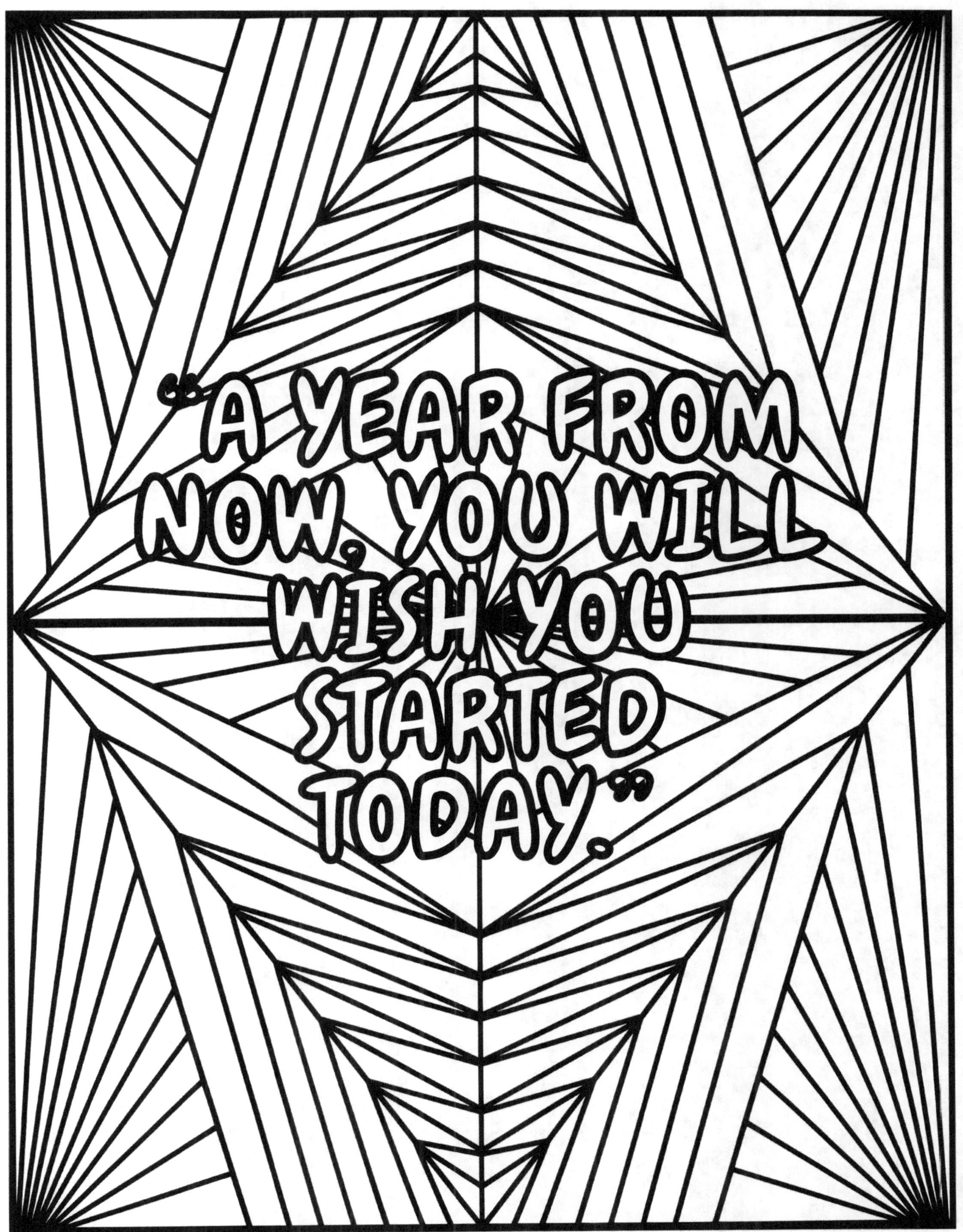

"A YEAR FROM NOW, YOU WILL WISH YOU STARTED TODAY."

"A year from now, you will wish
you started today."

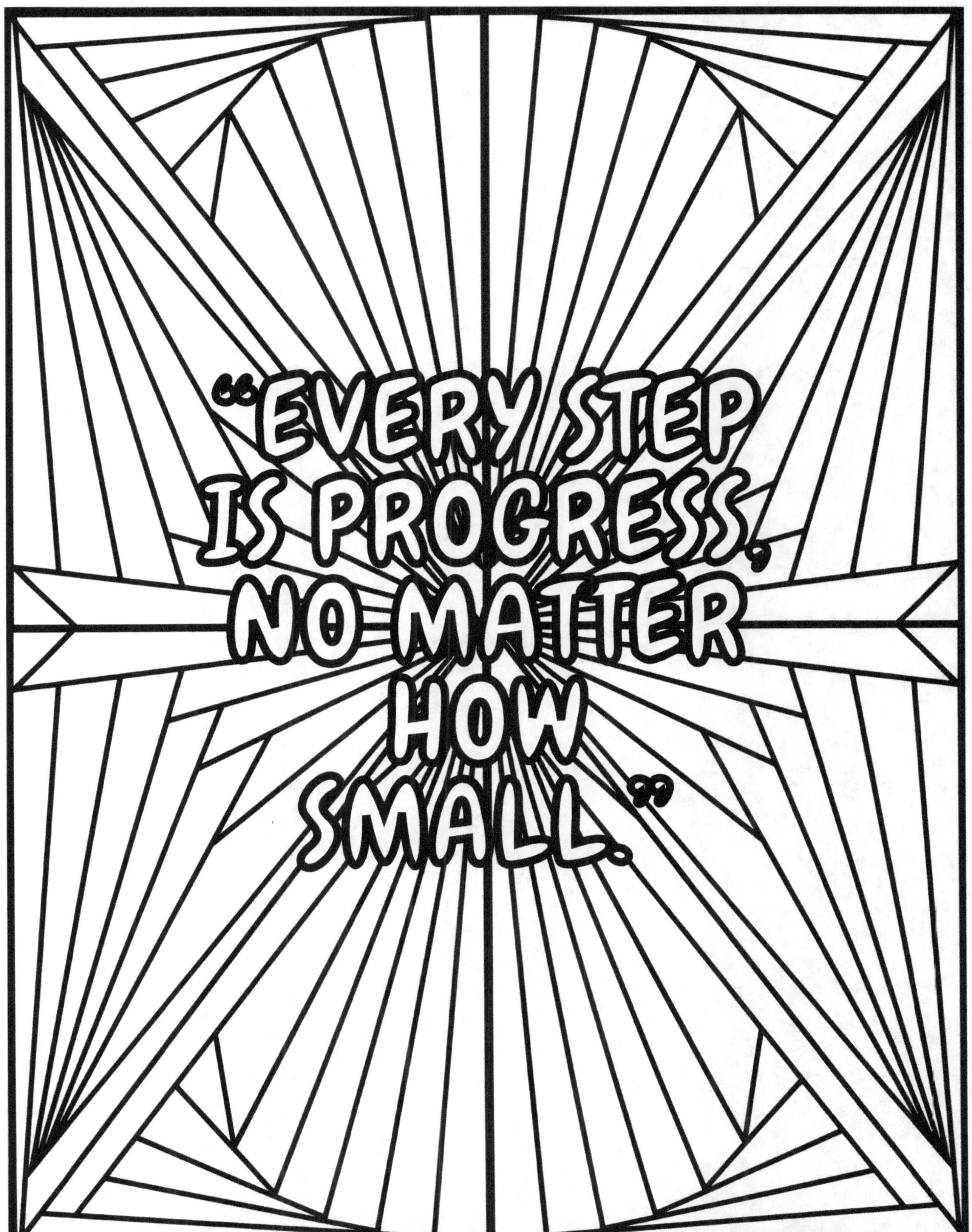

"EVERY STEP IS PROGRESS, NO MATTER HOW SMALL."

"Every step is progress, no matter how small."

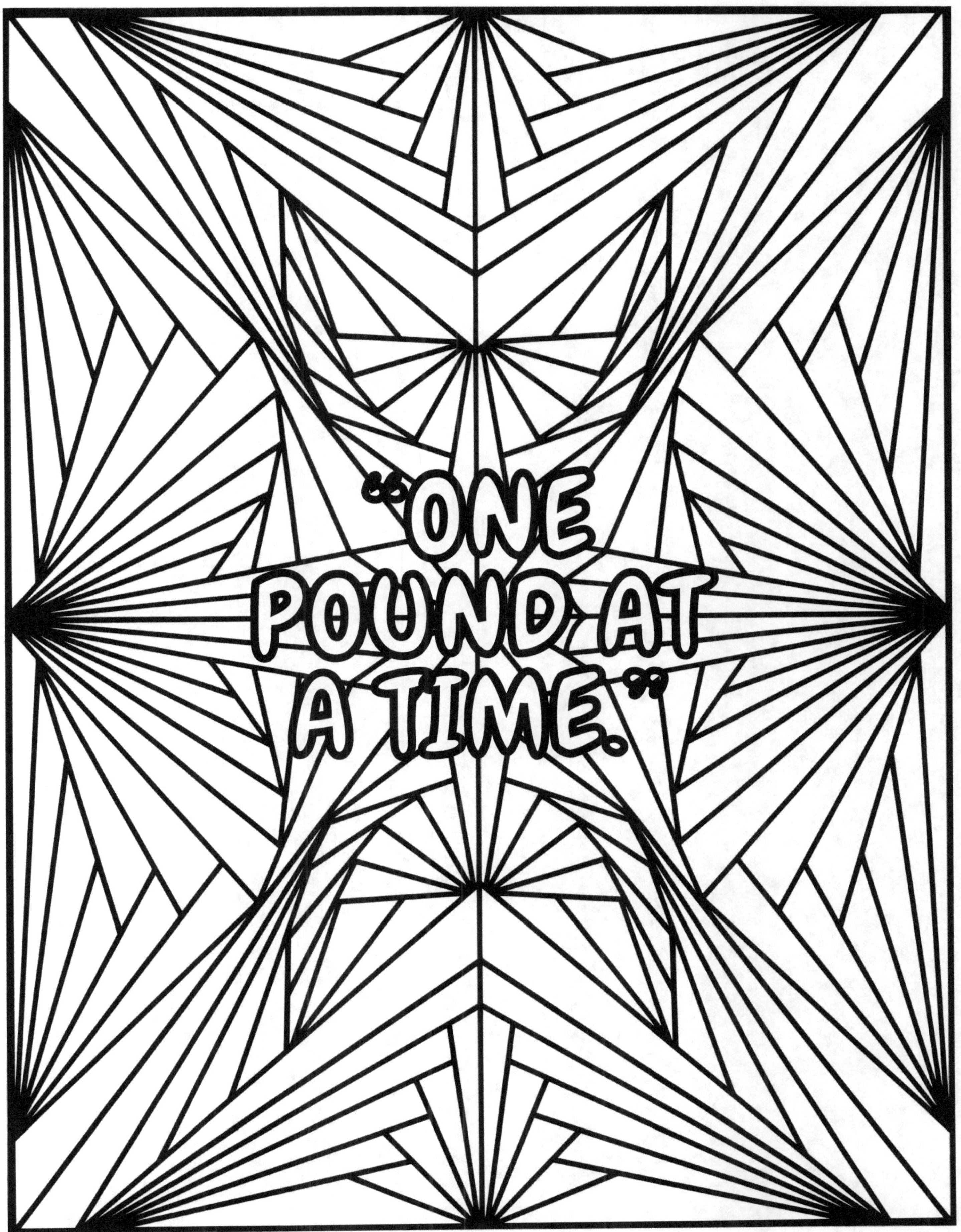
"ONE
POUND AT
A TIME."

"One pound at a time."

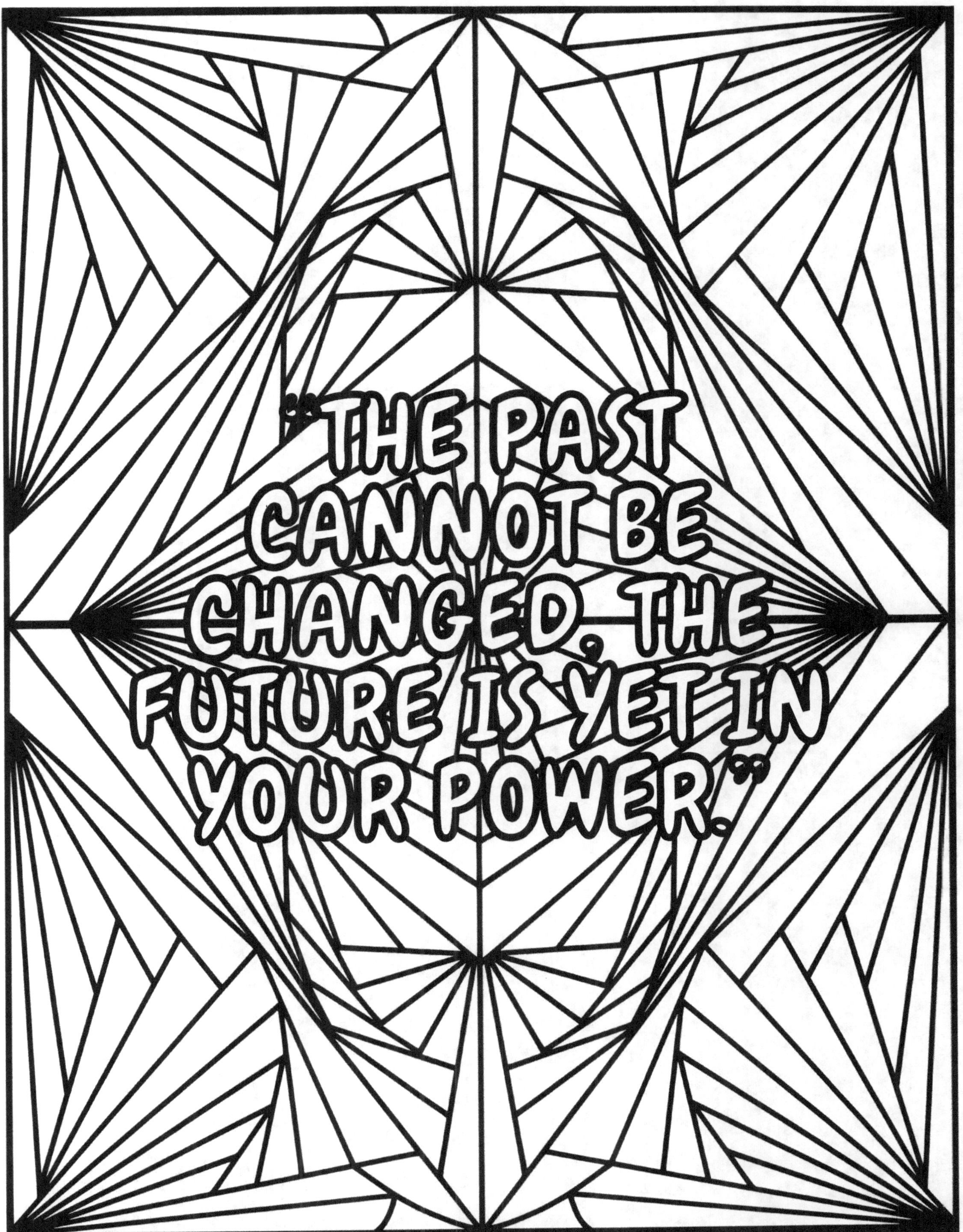

"THE PAST CANNOT BE CHANGED, THE FUTURE IS YET IN YOUR POWER."

"The past cannot be changed,
the future is yet in your power."

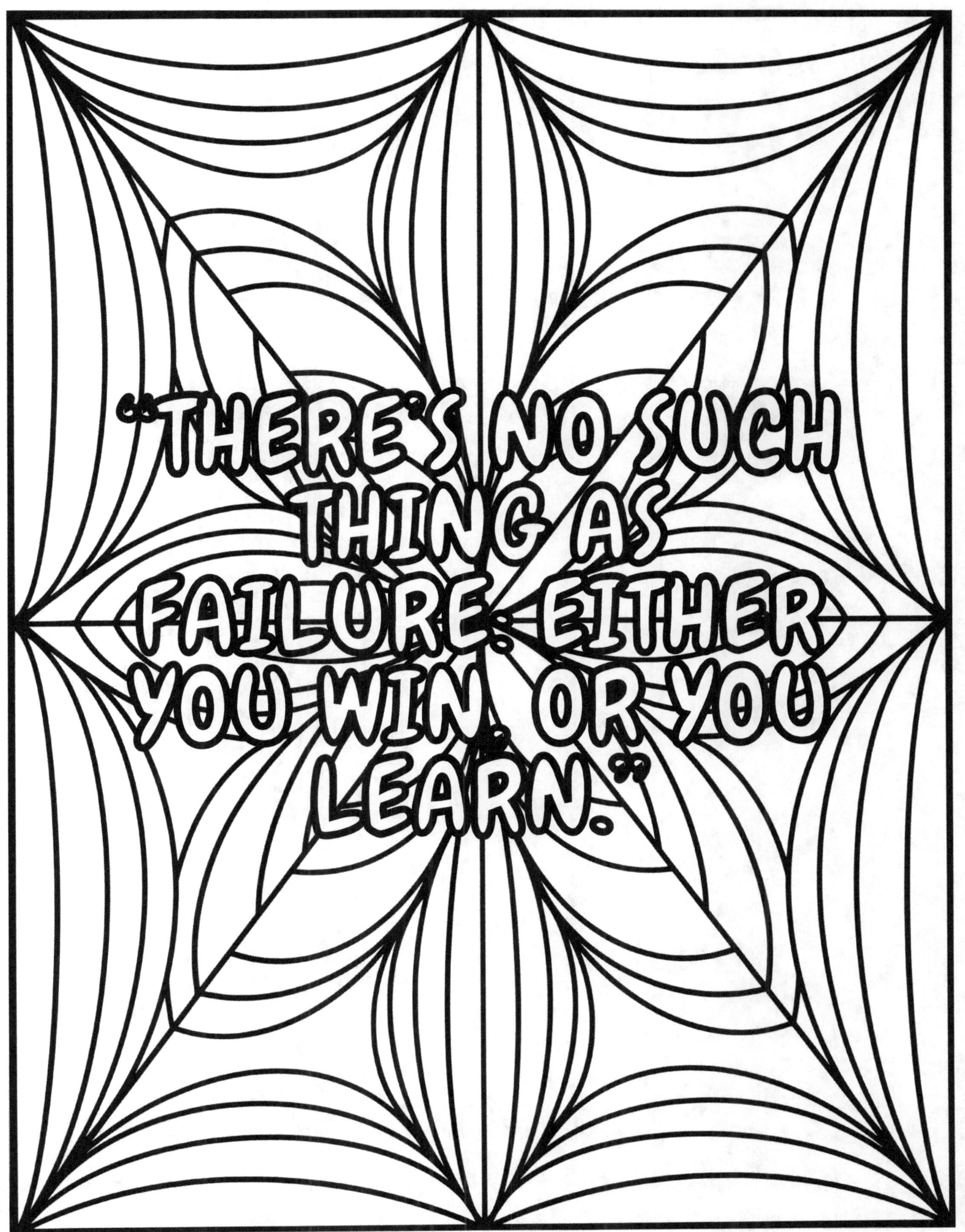

"THERE'S NO SUCH THING AS FAILURE. EITHER YOU WIN, OR YOU LEARN."

"There's no such thing as failure:
either you win, or you learn."

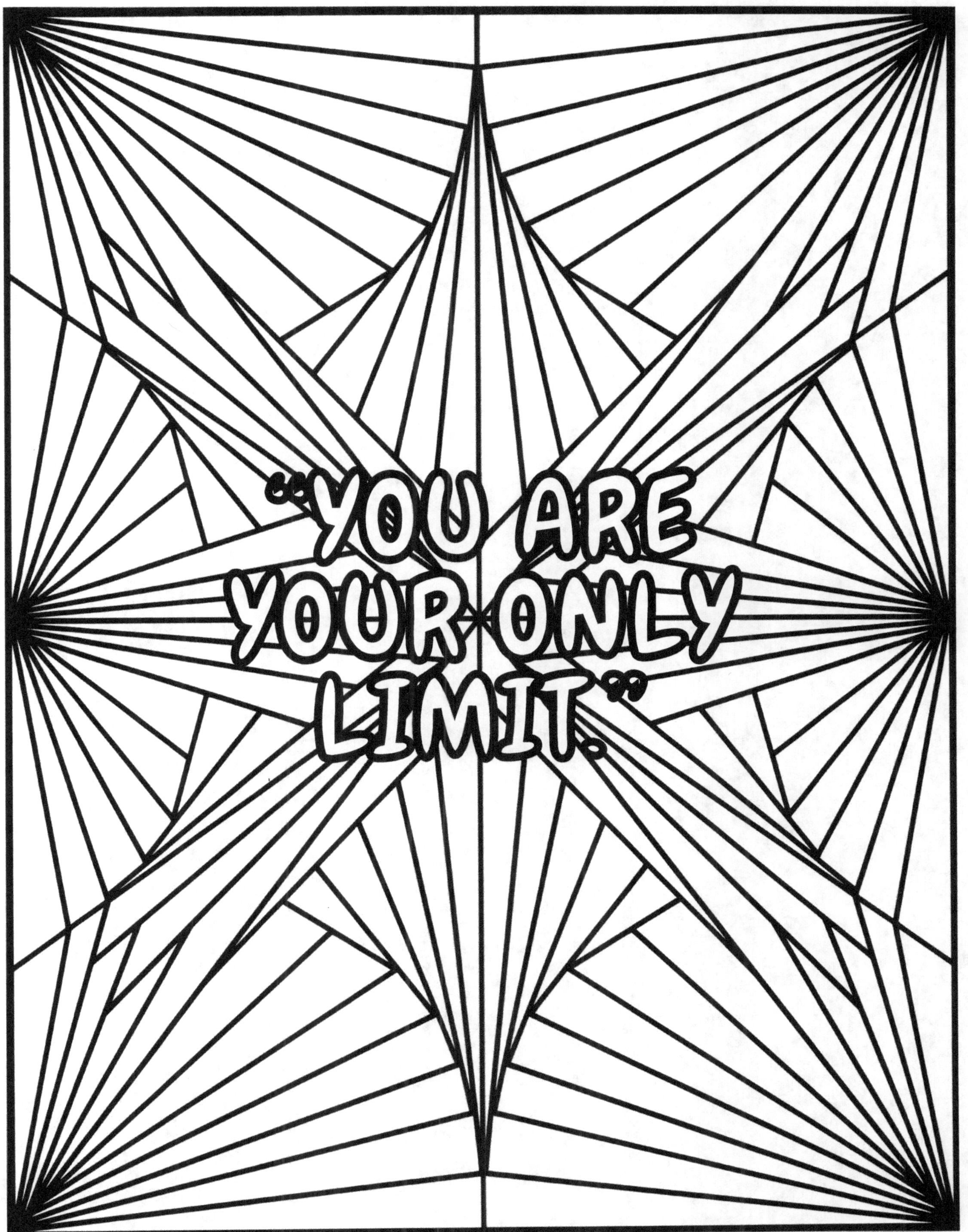

"YOU ARE YOUR ONLY LIMIT."

"You are your only limit."

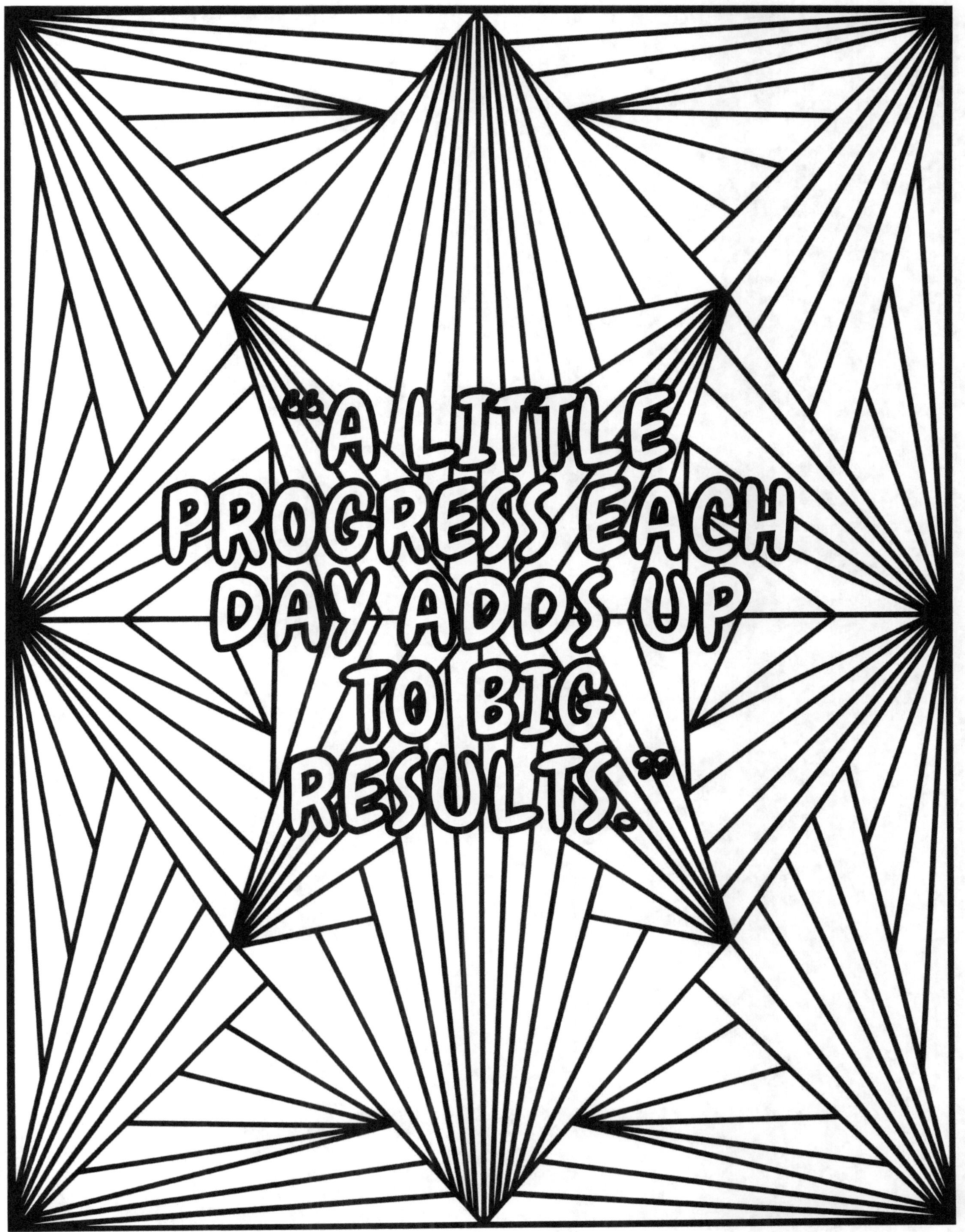
"A LITTLE PROGRESS EACH DAY ADDS UP TO BIG RESULTS."

"A little progress each day adds
up to big results."

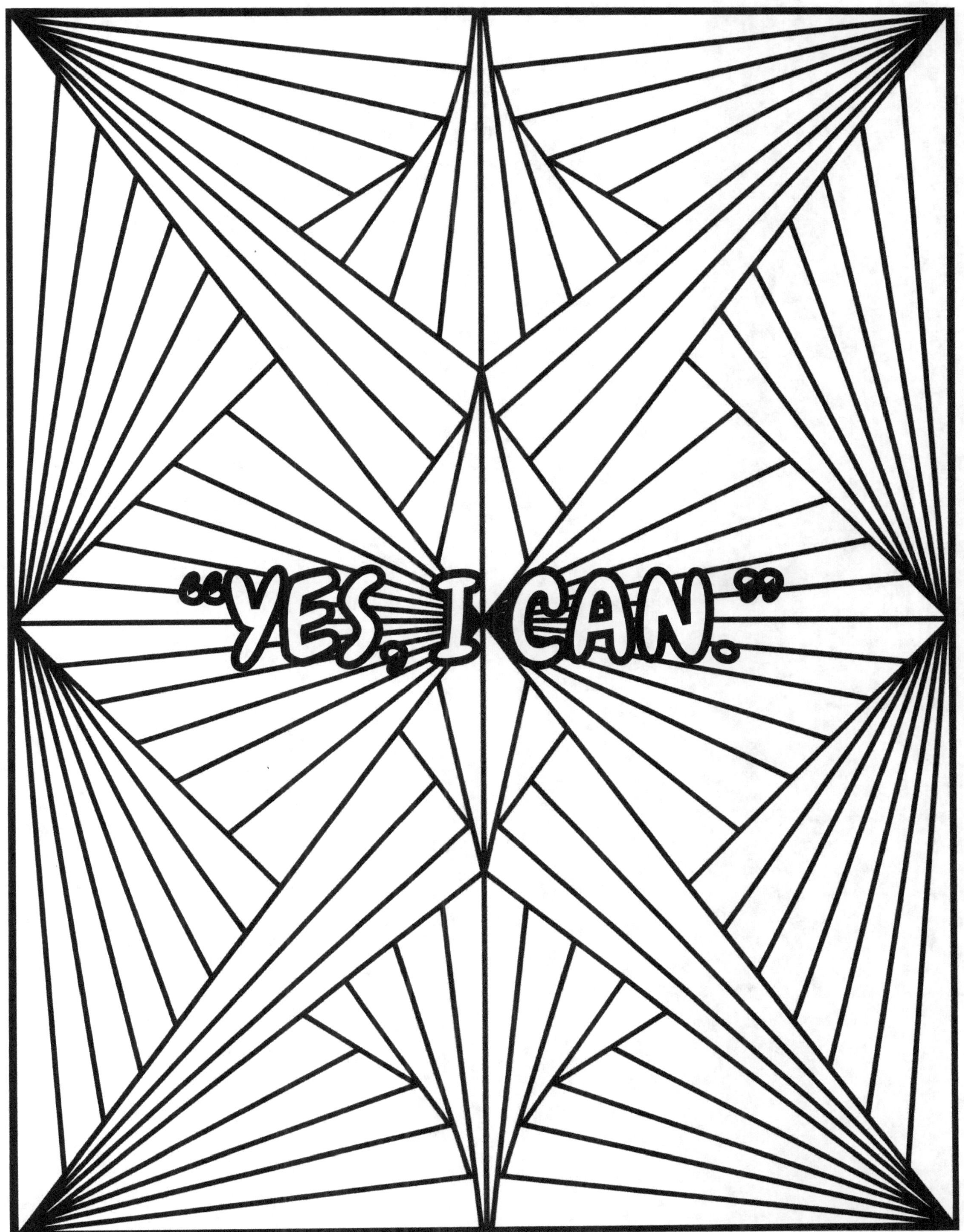

"YES, I CAN."

"Yes, I can."

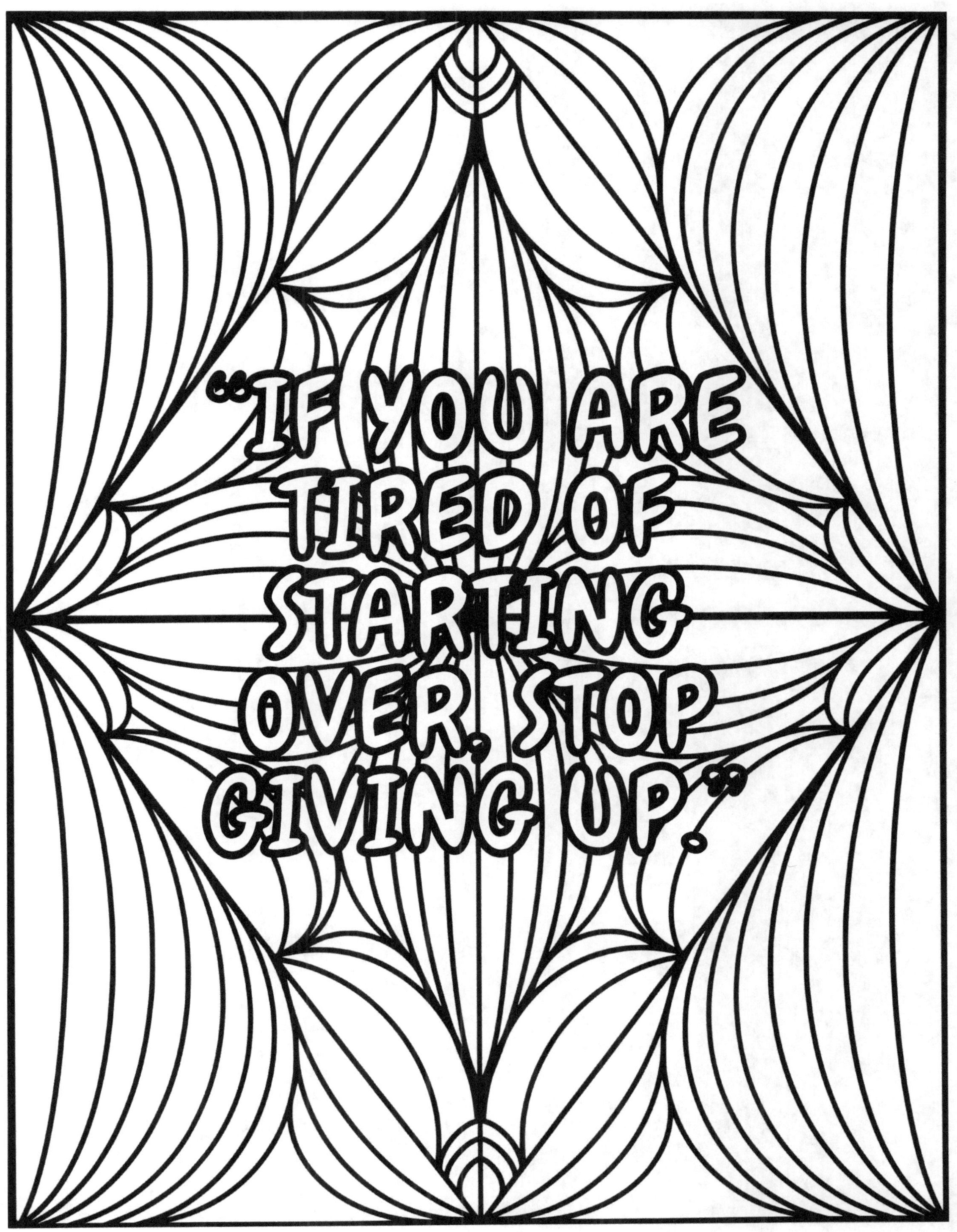
"IF YOU ARE TIRED OF STARTING OVER, STOP GIVING UP."

"If You Are Tired Of Starting Over,
Stop Giving Up."

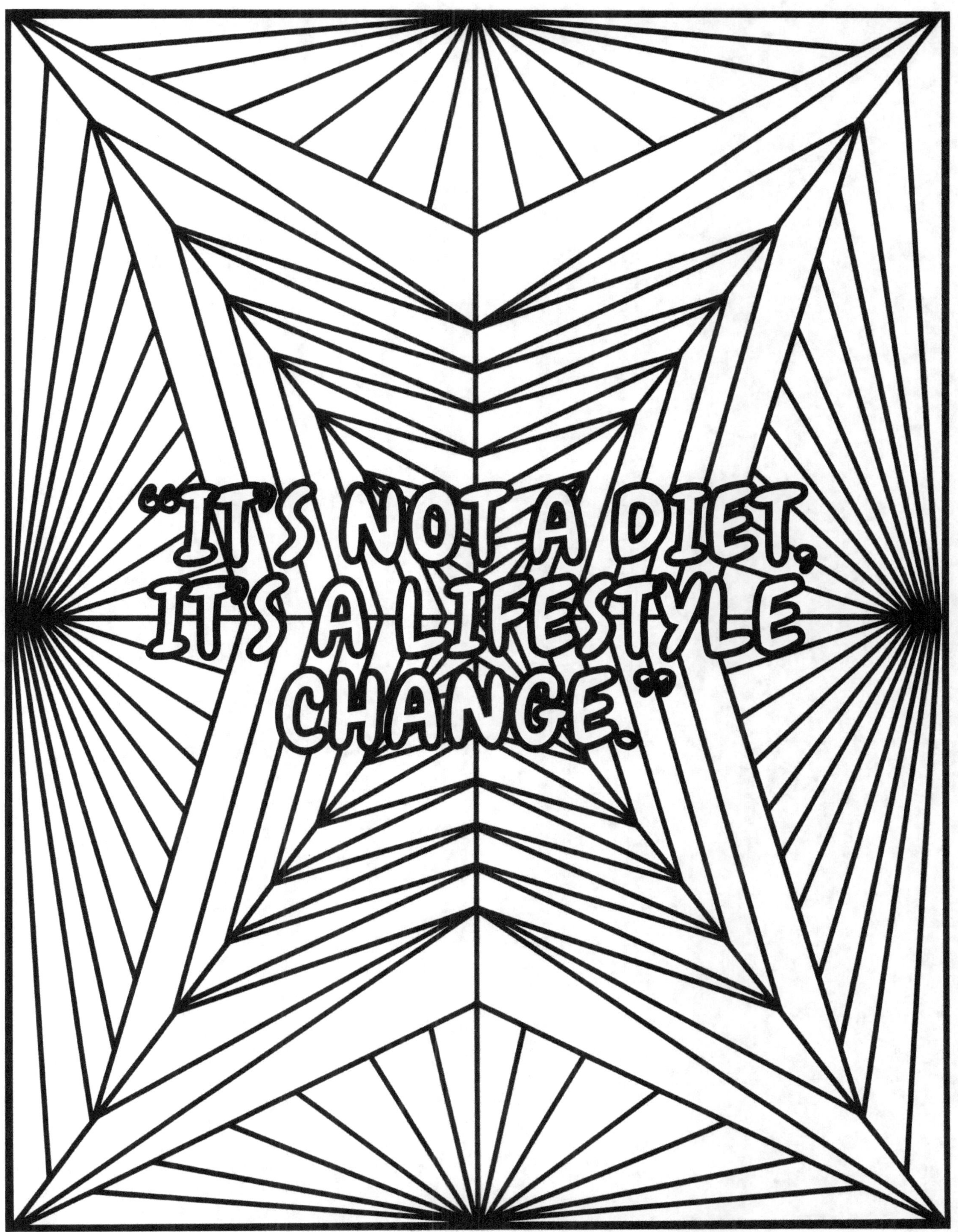

"IT'S NOT A DIET.
IT'S A LIFESTYLE
CHANGE."

"It's Not A Diet, It's A Lifestyle Change."

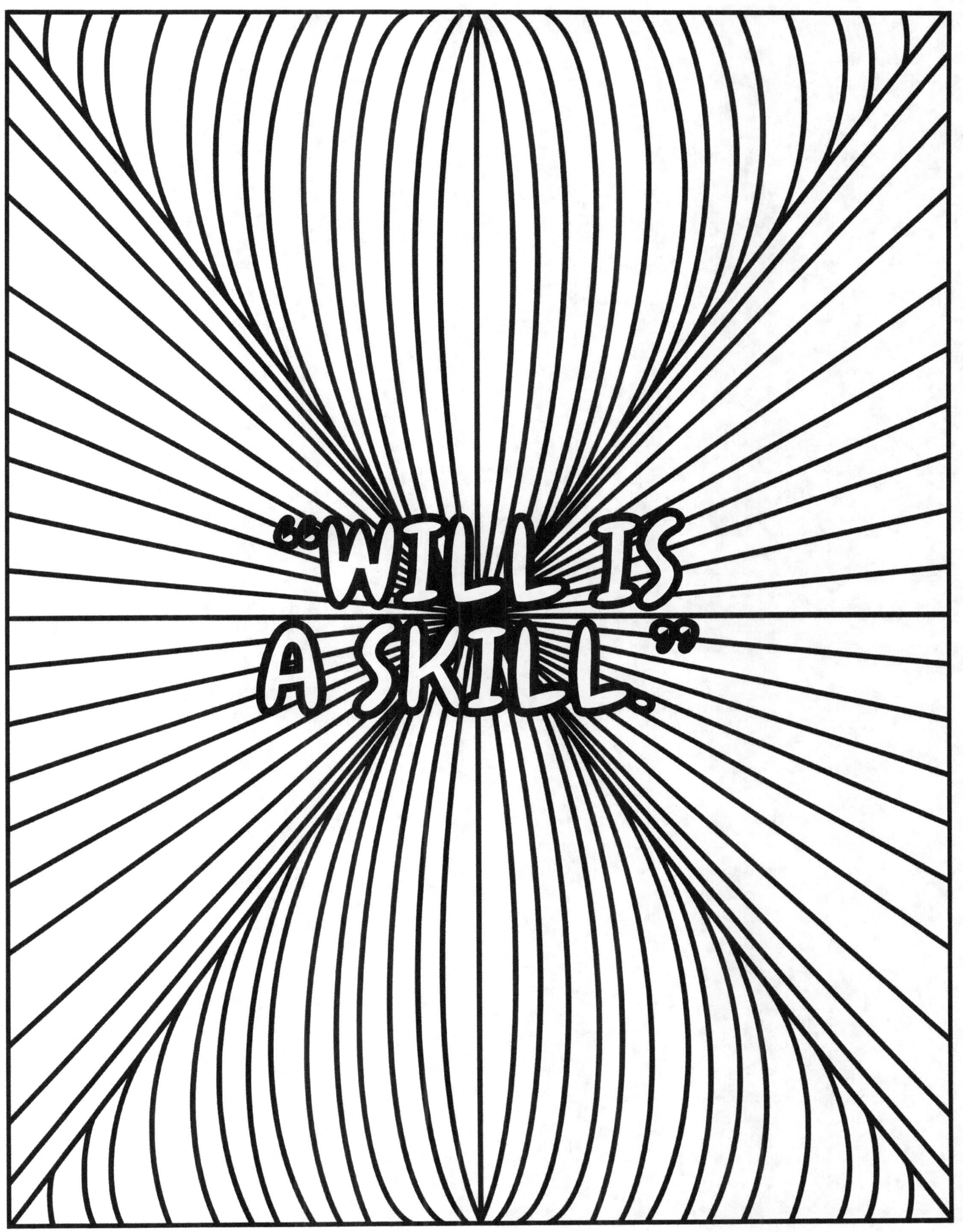

"WILL IS
A SKILL."

"Will Is A Skill."

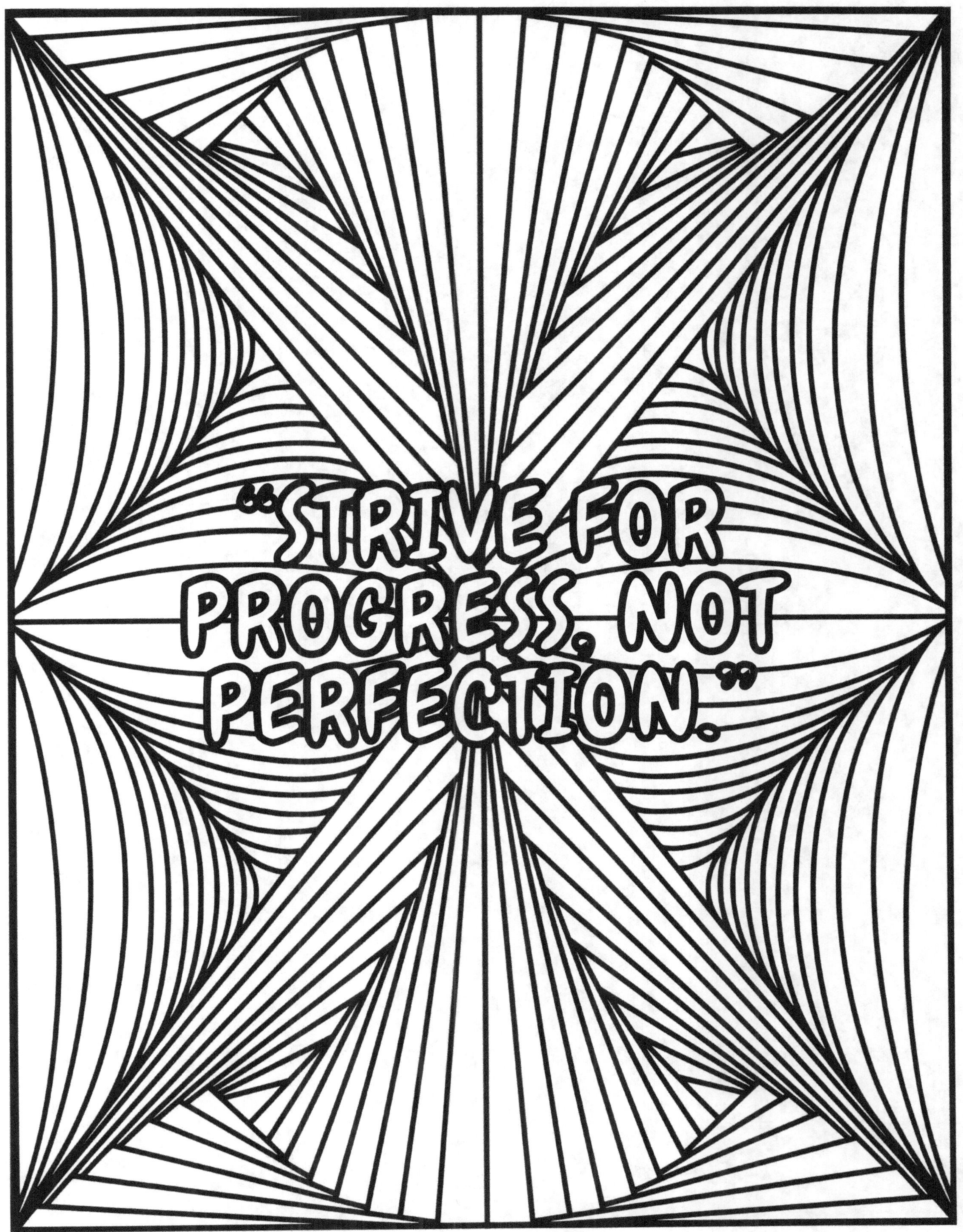
"STRIVE FOR PROGRESS, NOT PERFECTION."

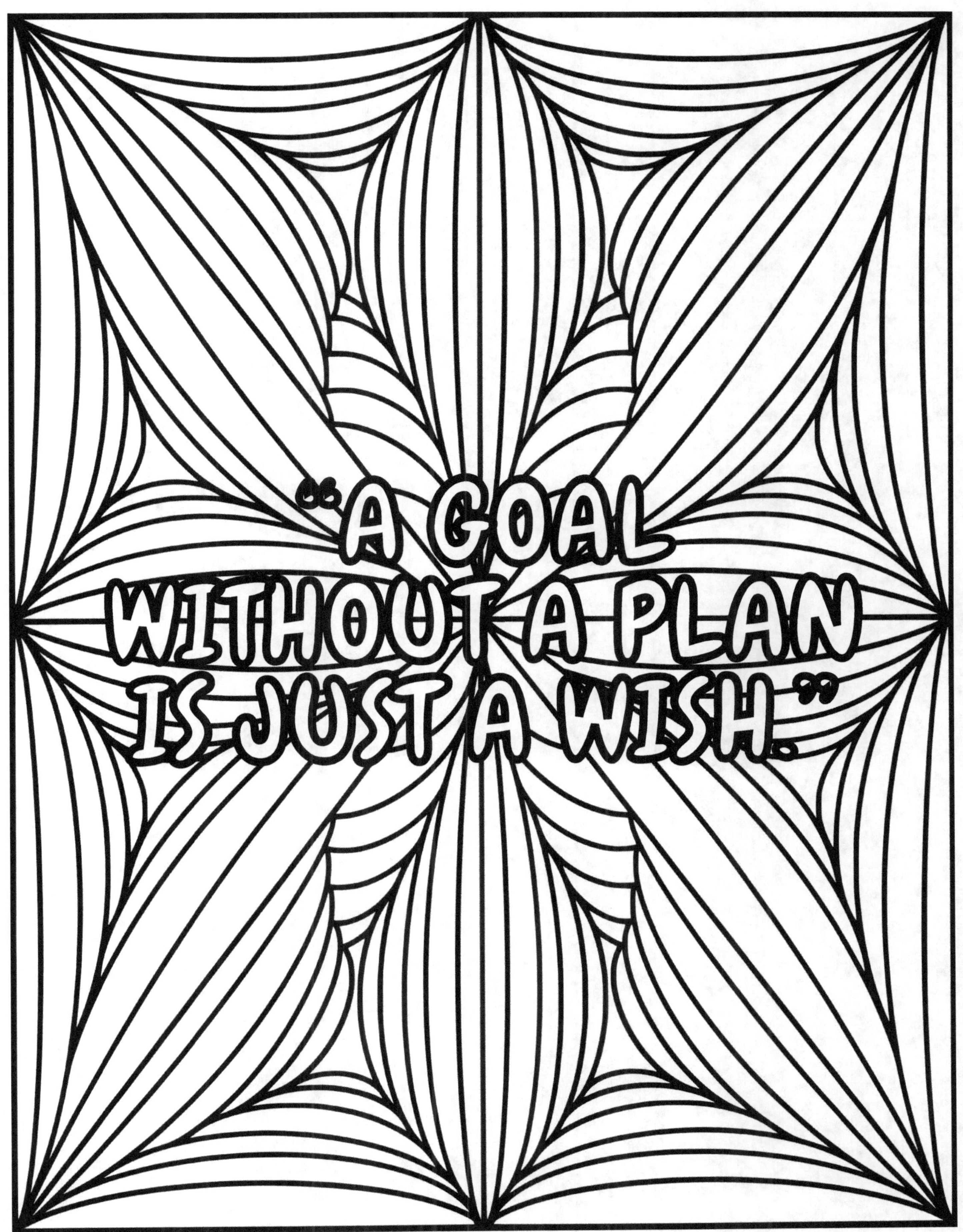

"A GOAL
WITHOUT A PLAN
IS JUST A WISH."

"A Goal Without A Plan Is Just A Wish."

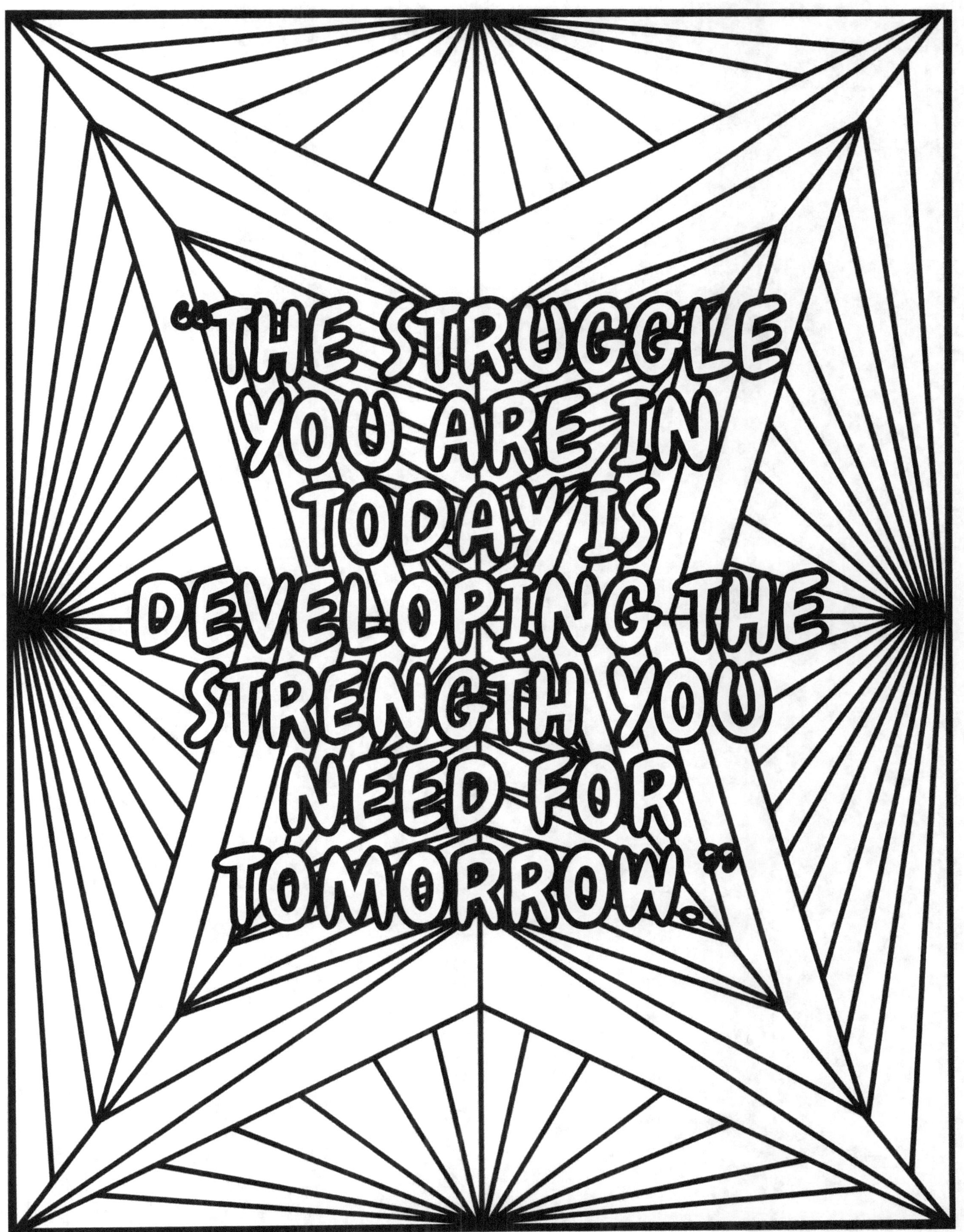

"THE STRUGGLE YOU ARE IN TODAY IS DEVELOPING THE STRENGTH YOU NEED FOR TOMORROW."

"The Struggle You Are In Today Is Developing The Strength You Need for Tomorrow."

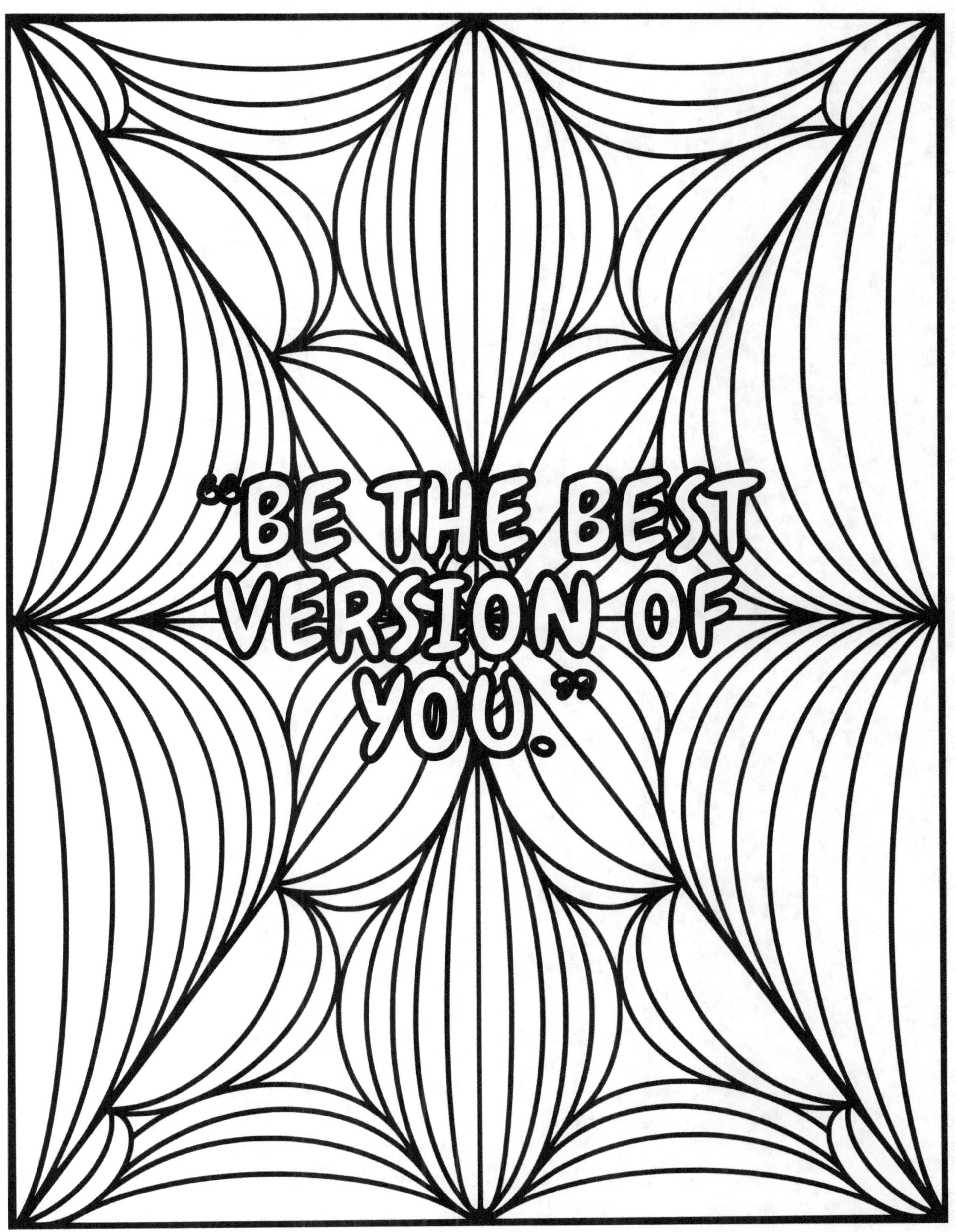

"BE THE BEST VERSION OF YOU."

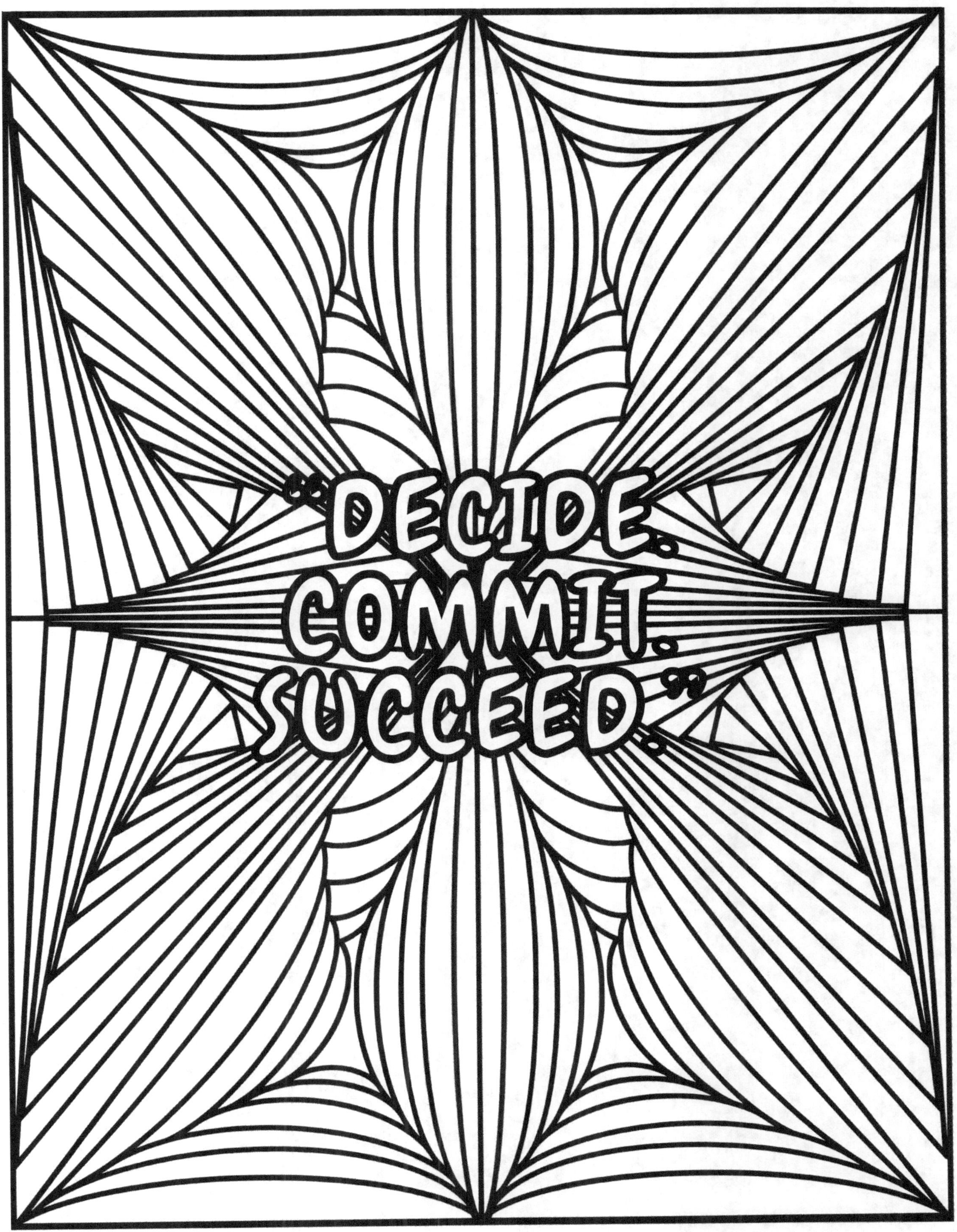

"DECIDE.
COMMIT.
SUCCEED."

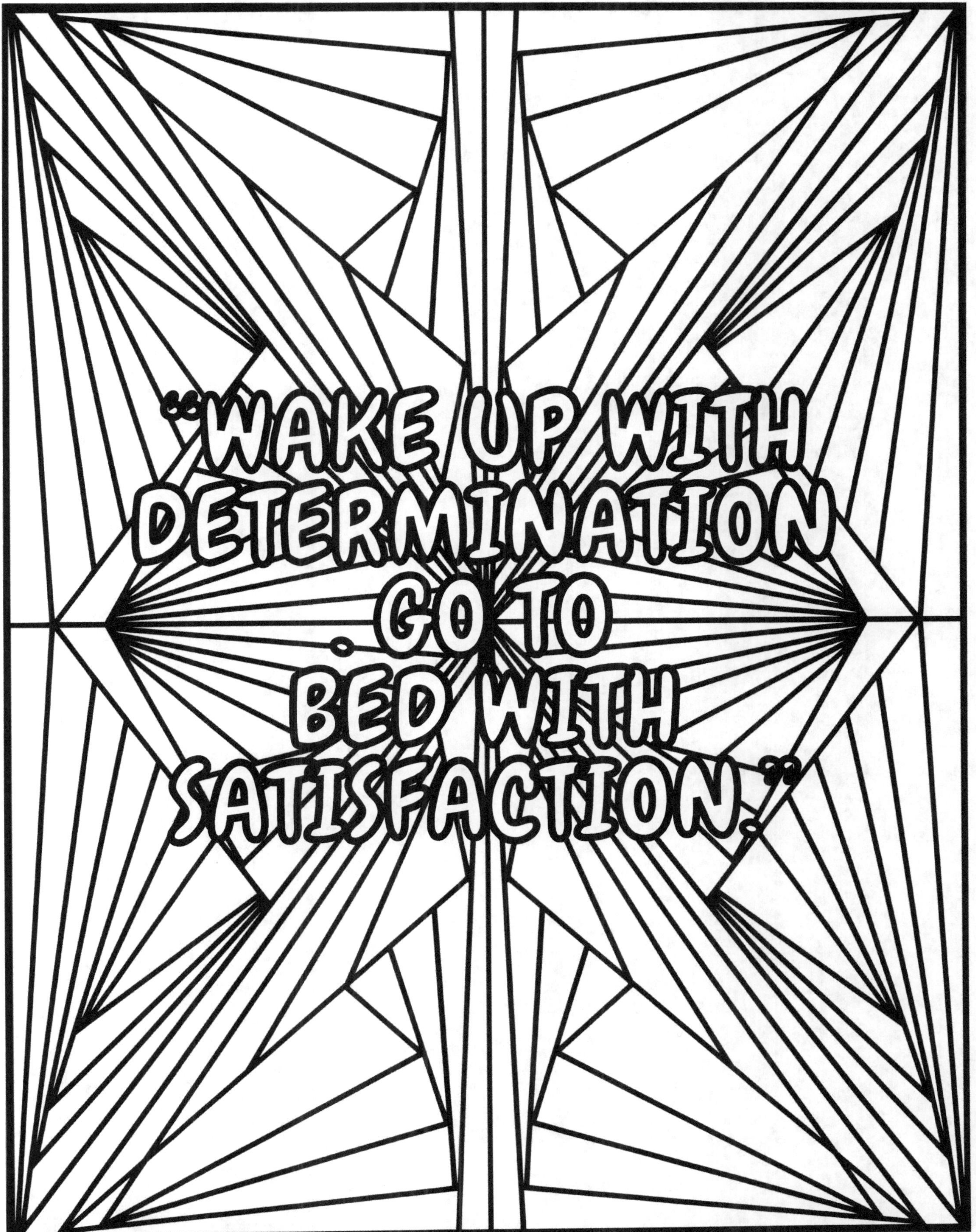

"WAKE UP WITH DETERMINATION GO TO BED WITH SATISFACTION."

"Wake up with determination. Go to
bed with satisfaction."

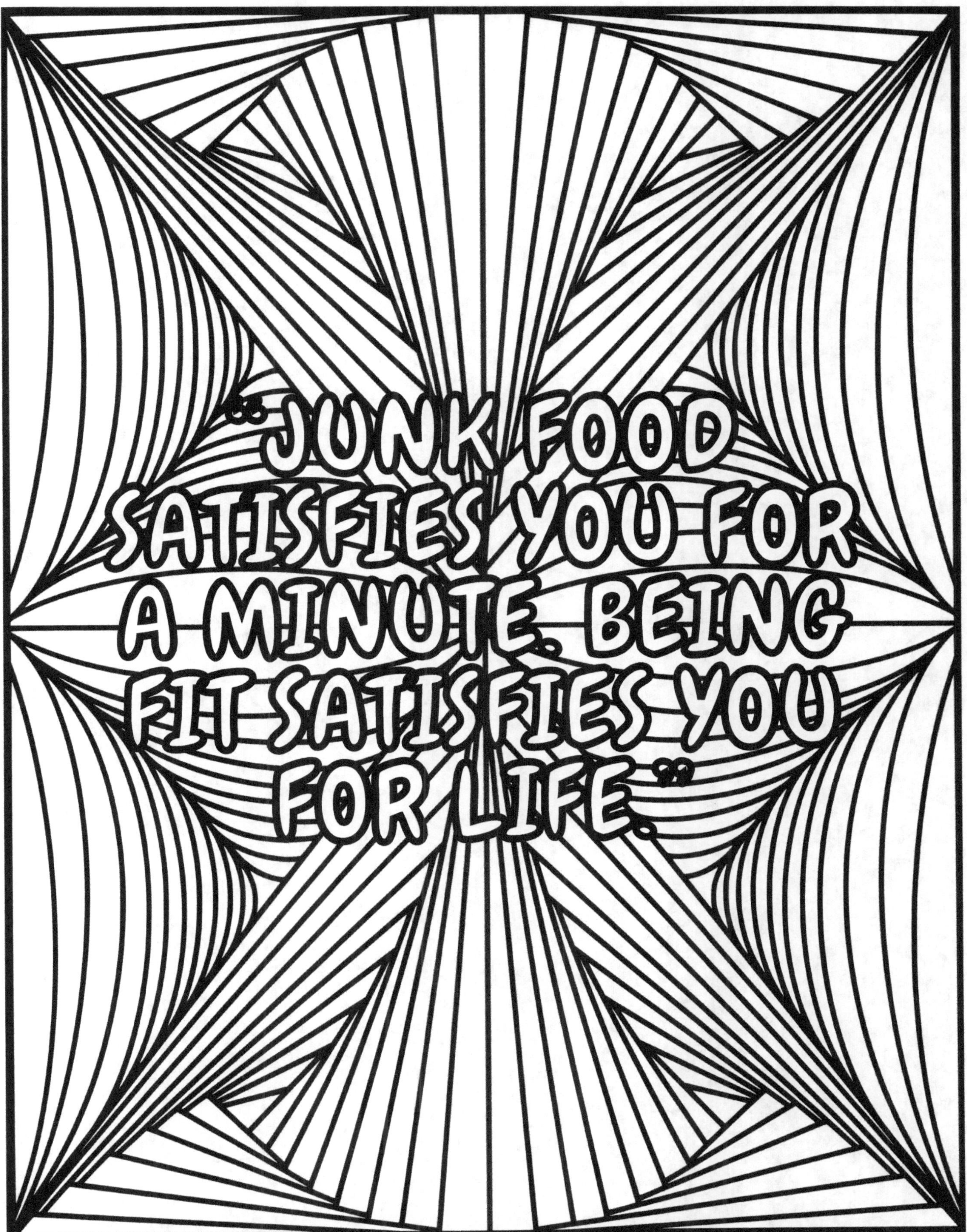

"JUNK FOOD SATISFIES YOU FOR A MINUTE. BEING FIT SATISFIES YOU FOR LIFE."

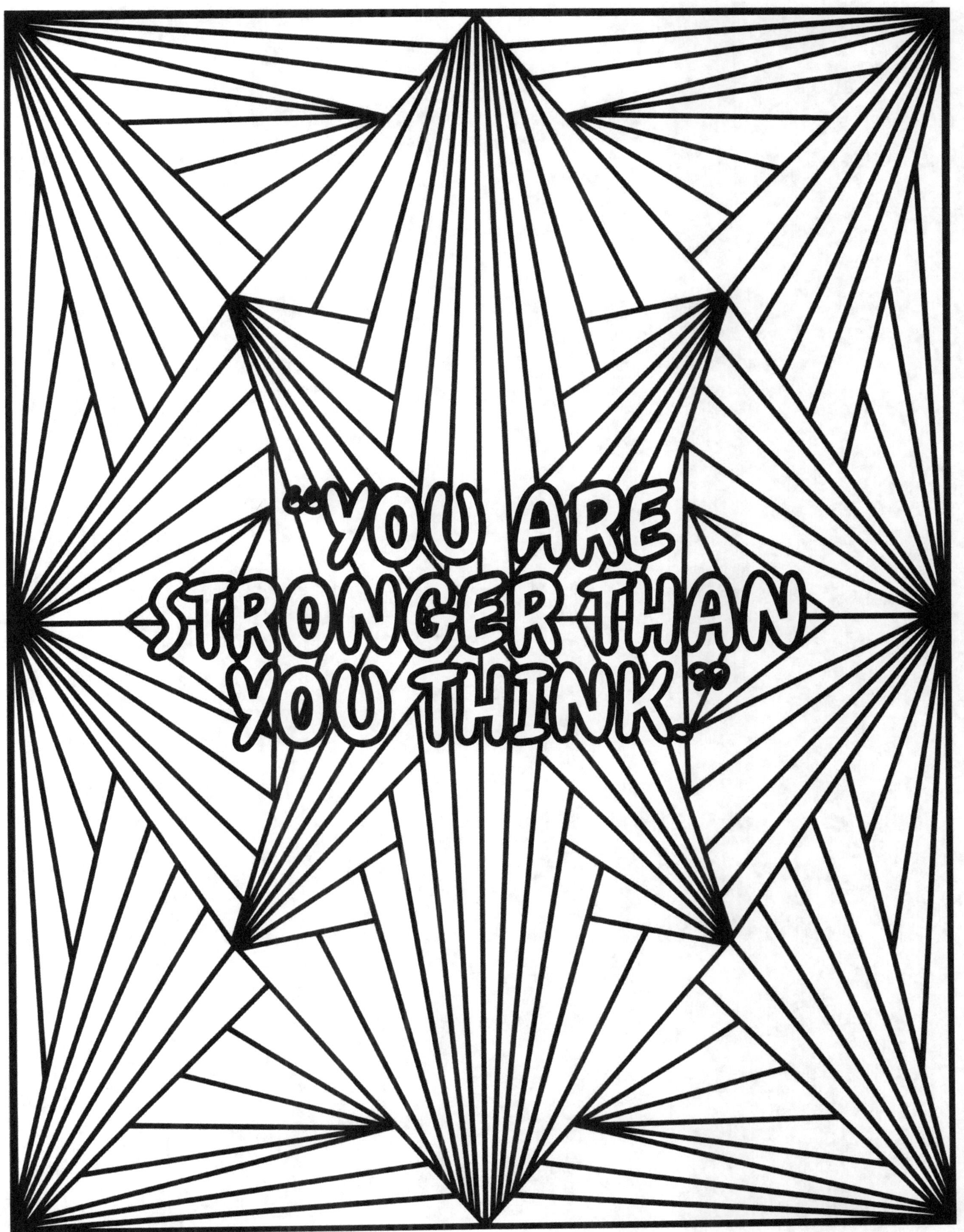

"YOU ARE STRONGER THAN YOU THINK."

"You are stronger than you think."

"You are stronger than you think."